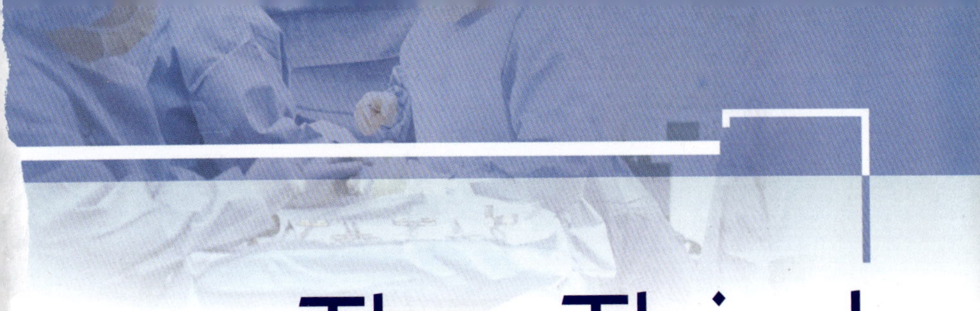

The Third Dimension of Surgery

The Third Dimension of Surgery

Sudarshan Nagaonkar
MTech (IIT, Bombay)
Director
Precious Life Medical Technologies Pvt Ltd.
Bengluru
email: ceo@preciouslife.co.in

Girish Gangan
MS (USA)
Director
Uma Surgicals Pvt Ltd.
Mumbai
email: girish@umasurgicals.com

CBSPD

CBS Publishers & Distributors Pvt Ltd

New Delhi • Bengaluru • Chennai • Kochi • Kolkata • Lucknow • Mumbai
Hyderabad • Jharkhand • Nagpur • Patna • Pune • Uttarakhand

Disclaimer

Science and technology are constantly changing fields. New research and experience broaden the scope of information and knowledge. The authors have tried their best in giving information available to them while preparing the material for this book. Although all efforts have been made to ensure optimum accuracy of the material, yet it is quite possible some errors might have been left uncorrected. The publisher, the printer, and the authors will not be held responsible for any inadvertent errors or inaccuracies.

The Third Dimension of Surgery

ISBN: 978-93-5466-763-3

First Edition: 2024

Published by Satish Kumar Jain and produced by Varun Jain for

CBS Publishers & Distributors Pvt Ltd

4819/XI Prahlad Street, 24 Ansari Road, Daryaganj, New Delhi 110 002, India

Ph: 011-23289259, 23266861 e-mail: delhi@cbspd.com Website: www.cbspd.com

Corporate Office: 204 FIE, Industrial Area, Patparganj, Delhi 110 092, India

Ph: 011-49344934 Fax: 011-49344935 e-mail: publishing@cbspd.com; publicity@cbspd.com

Branches

- **Bengaluru:** Seema House 2975, 17th Cross, KR Road, Banasankari 2nd Stage, Bengaluru 560 070, Karnataka, India
  Ph: +91-80-26771678/79 Fax: +91-80-26771680 e-mail: bangalore@cbspd.com
- **Chennai:** 7, Subbaraya Street, Shenoy Nagar, Chennai 600 030, Tamil Nadu, India
  Ph: +91-44-26680620, 26681266 Fax: +91-44-42032115 e-mail: chennai@cbspd.com
- **Kochi:** 42/1325, 1326, Power House Road, Opposite KSEB, Power House, Ernakulam 682 018, Kochi, Kerala, India
  Ph: +91-484-4059061–67 Fax: +91-484-4059065 e-mail: kochi@cbspd.com
- **Kolkata:** 147, Hind Ceramics Compound, 1st Floor, Nilgunj Road, Belghoria, Kolkata 700 056, West Bengal, India
  Ph: +91-33-25330055/56 e-mail: kolkata@cbspd.com
- **Lucknow:** Basement, Khushnuma Complex, 7 Meerabai Marg (behind Jawahar Bhawan), Lucknow 226 001, UP, India
  Ph: +91-522-4000032 e-mail: tiwari.lucknow@cbspd.com
- **Mumbai:** PWD Shed, Gala No. 25/26, Ramchandra Bhatt Marg, Next JJ Hospital Gate No. 2, Opp. Union Bank of India, Noorbaug, Mumbai 400 009, Maharashtra, India
  Ph: +91-22-66661880/89 e-mail: mumbai@cbspd.com

Representatives

- **Hyderabad** 0-9885175004
- **Jharkhand** 0-9811541605
- **Nagpur** 0-8692091830
- **Patna** 0-9334159340
- **Pune** 0-9664372571
- **Uttarakhand** 0-9716462459

Printed at: Gokul Offset Pvt. Ltd, Delhi, India.

Foreword

It is my pleasure to introduce you *The Third Dimension of Surgery*. This book is a comprehensive guide to the technological advancements in the field of surgery, starting with the most common technologies like energy sources to the most promising technologies in the field.

The book is divided into six chapters, each of which focuses on a specific technology, the fundamental concepts and its applications in surgery. The book is authored by an expert in this field, who has provided a detailed overview of the technology, its current state of development and potential impact on the future of surgery.

Being a surgeon and as an interested person in the technological aspects in the field of surgery, I am particularly excited about the potential of these technologies to revolutionise the field. From robot-assisted surgery to 3D printing, these technologies have the potential to improve patient outcomes, reduce complications, and make surgery safer and more efficient.

I hope that this book will serve as a valuable resource for anyone who is interested in learning about the latest technological advancements in surgery. I would like to thank Mr Sudarshan for his sincere contribution and effort to this book, and I hope that entire surgical fraternity finds it informative and engaging.

Prof Tamonas Chaudhuri
MBBS, MS. FAIS, FMAS, FACS

Professor
Department of Surgery
Burdwan Medical College
Purba Bardhaman, West Bengal, India

Consultant
ILS Hospitals, Kolkata
West Bengal, India

Preface

Congratulations on buying this book. This shows your commitment to learning about technologies related to surgery and you have already separated yourself from others.

Success in surgery depends on understanding of anatomy, surgical hand and the technology. Anatomy is mastered by the surgeons as part of their graduate and postgraduate studies; the surgical hand gets better with practice. It is the technology part that is less emphasised even though its role in surgery is expanding ever. This book exclusively focuses on the technology aspect of surgery and that is why title of the book is *The Third Dimension of Surgery*.

This book has been written for surgeons to help them in two ways viz. (i) when they buy a technology product, they are better equipped to have meaningful discussion with the vendors and select the right product for them and (ii) use their technology assets in safe and effective manner. The practicing surgeons can use this book as a reference to understand a specific technology deeper either because of an impending buying decision or the need to train their staff on a specific topic is felt.

This book is also useful to the postgraduate students, to get them headstart in surgery technology domain. They will be able to apply this understanding during their postgraduation and also start their surgery practice on a more sound footing.

Some biomedical engineers may find this book useful. This book is recommended to them only after they have some exposure to surgery, and they have keen interest in a particular product.

The first two chapters cover energy sources, which is probably the most important piece of technology in the surgeon's life. The chapters cover electrosurgery, including monopolar, bipolar, vessel sealer, saline bipolar, ultrasonic scalpel and laser.

The third chapter covers medical lighting with special emphasis on OT light.

The fourth chapter covers medical optics. It covers laparoscopic camera, medical grade monitors and other related technologies for vision.

The fifth chapter covers the role of metals in surgery. This chapter covers the metallurgy in surgery, types of surgical instruments, selection criteria for instruments, tips for effective use of them and storage and handling instructions.

The sixth chapter covers the upcoming technologies, which are likely to have big impact on practice of surgery in the next few decades. The chapter covers robotic surgery, artificial intelligence with emphasis on machine learning, virtual reality, augmented reality and 3D printing.

Each chapter gets the reader familiar with the basic terms, explains the fundamental technology concepts, covers the practical tips for safe and effective surgery. Some chapters also have basic troubleshooting guide for some common problems.

The book is intended to become more practical than academic. Hence, simplicity has been prioritised against technical accuracy.

I am thankful to all the professionals from whom I have learnt these concepts and there are too many to enumerate. If the book has come out well, the credit goes to them. If there are errors or scope for improvement, those are because of my limitations. Please bring them to my notice and I will try to improve the content in the next edition.

My heartfelt thanks to my family members, who supported me in my pursuit of knowledge at the cost of family time. I thank Vibhor Anand for suggesting the book title. I also thank the Society of American Gastrointestinal and Endoscopic Surgeons (SAGES) for lightening the quest for knowledge in me.

Sudarshan Nagaonkar

Contents

3. Medical Lighting 37

4. Medical Optics 47

CHAPTER

1

Electrosurgery

Sudarshan Nagaonkar

Among all the energy sources, electrosurgery is the most commonly used energy source during surgery. Mastery of this will significantly reduce surgery time, cause less blood loss, have faster recovery for the patient and reduce the number of safety hazards.

In this chapter, we will cover the fundamentals of this technology, get you familiar with the terms used commonly related to this technology, discuss the dos and don'ts and some basic troubleshooting techniques.

Energy

Energy is ability to do work and it is measured in Joules. **Power**, measured in watts, denotes the rate of delivery of energy. In most cases, the energy is converted from one form to another, e.g. flow of current (electrical energy) through any material causes generation of heat (heat energy) in it. Geysers and electric heaters use this principle.

Current is flow of electrons. Current is measured at a cross section and the unit of measurement is amperes. Flow of current is caused by potential difference between two points. That potential difference is voltage. Voltage is measured between two points and the unit of measurement is volts. The characteristic of material which opposes flow of current is called as resistance or Impedance. The impedance is measured between two points and the unit of measurement is ohm.

Ohms law says that

Current (I) = Voltage (V)/Impedance (R).

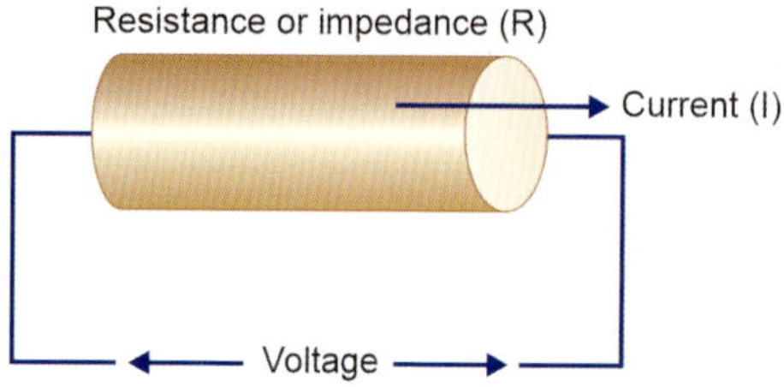

Fig. 1.1: Ohm's law

As seen in Fig. 1.1, an electrical circuit will have voltage, current and impedance. The relationship among these parameters is stated by Ohm's law.

Also, Power (W) = Voltage (V) × Current (I).

Now that we have covered basic physics terms, let's understand fundamentals of electrosurgery.

Electrosurgery

Electrosurgery is a technology that is used for cutting and coagulation effects by passing current through the patient tissue and thereby elevating temperature of the tissue for the desired effect. It has mainly two modes viz. *monopolar* and *bipolar*. The electrosurgery converts electrical energy into heat energy in a controlled manner to get the desired effect.

Monopolar Mode

Monopolar is a mode within electrosurgery which utilises combination of the instrument and dispersive electrode aka patient plate for completing the current path.

In monopolar mode, the current path is, as depicted in Fig. 1.2, as follows:

- Electrosurgical generator
- Electrode at the site of surgery
- Patient body
- Dispersive electrode
- Electrosurgical generator.

It is important to note that the amount of current flowing through the electrode and the dispersive electrode is exactly the same. We get effect on the tissue at the site of surgery because

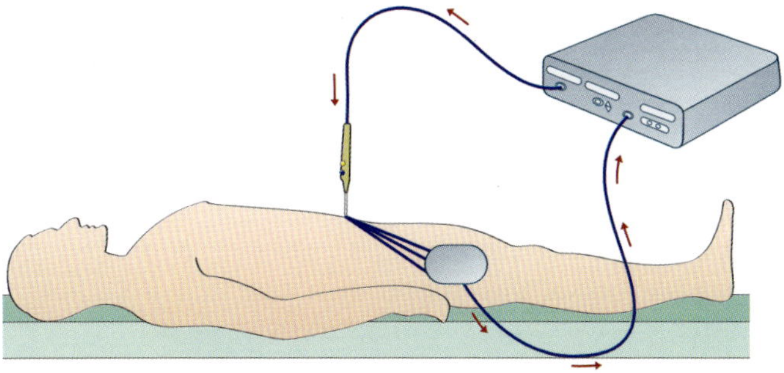

Fig. 1.2: Monopolar mode of electrosurgery

the current is concentrated and hardly any temerature elevation at the dispersive electrode because the current spread over a large area.

Since this has safety implication, let me elaborate this point further:

As shown in Fig. 1.3, when we place a piece of paper in the sunlight, it does not burn. However, when we concentrate the sunlight using a lens, it has the capability to burn it.

This is exacly what happens while using monopolar. The energy is concentrated at the electrode while it is dispersed at the dispersive electrode.

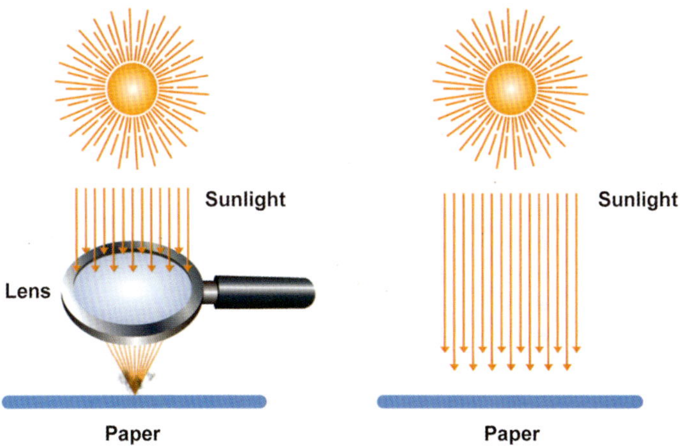

Fig. 1.3: Concentration of energy v/s dispersion of energy

Bipolar Mode

Biopolar is a mode within electrosurgery which utilises electrodes within the instrument for completing the current path.

In bipolar mode, as depicted in Fig. 1.4, the current path is as follows:

- Electrosurgical generator
- One electrode of the bipolar instrument
- Another electrode of the bipolar instrument
- Electrosurgical generator.

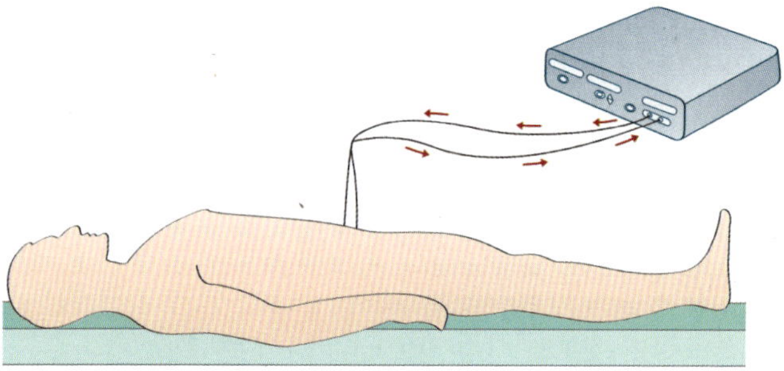

Fig. 1.4: Bipolar mode of electrosurgery

It is important to note that bipolar does not require dispersive electrode.

Vessel sealer and saline bipolar are special modes under the overall umbrella of bipolar modes.

Effect of Frequency on the Tissue

The regular power supply in our homes and offices can cause electrocution. However, the electrosurgery current causes only heat generation in the patient tissue. The difference is in the operating frequencies.

The mains supply has operating frequency of 50 Hz. These are typically known as low frequency, as depicted in Fig. 1.5. At this frequency, there can be neuromuscular stimulation. However, electrosurgery uses frequency of above 100 kHz, typically between 300 kHz and 700 kHz. These are high frequency, as depicted in Fig. 1.5. That is the reason the electrosurgery does not cause any neuromuscular stimulation.

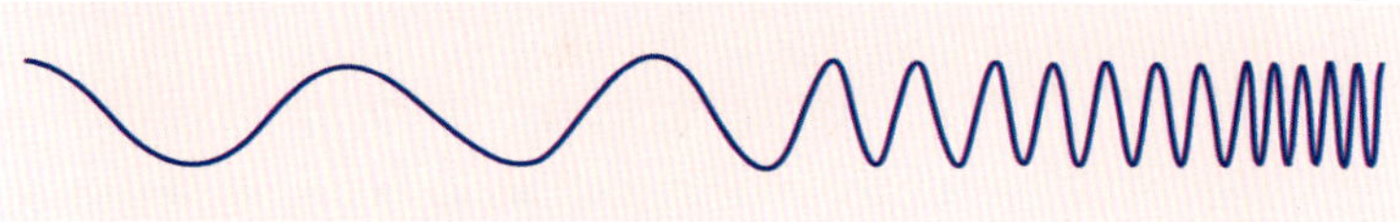

Fig. 1.5: Range of frequencies

Effect of Temperature Rise on the Tissue

There are various effects on the tissue as a response to heating. The temperature ranges and the corresponding effects are given in Table 1.1.

Table 1.1: Effect of temperature rise on the tissue

Temperature	*Effect on tissue*
<50°	Reversible changes in tissue
52° for >6 minutes	Irreversible change starts
60–80°	Desiccation and protein denaturation
120°	Tissue evaporation
>200°	Tissue charring

For temperatures below 50 degrees, there will be changes in the tissue like reducing water content. However, these changes are reversible and the body will replenish the water content.

For temperatures above 52 degrees for more than 6 minutes, irreversible changes start happening.

For temperatures between 60 and 80 degrees, two changes happen:

1. The water content in the cells reduces and the cells dry, know as desiccation.
2. The protein content of the cells gets denatured, i.e. protein gets converted from liquid to solid and changes its colour from colourless to white.

These two effects can be seen in Fig. 1.6.

The combined effect desiccation and protein denaturation is that the capillaries get blocked and thus coagulation is achieved.

For temperatures above 100 degrees and around 120 degrees, the water content of the cells start boiling, which causes cell evapouration, which causes cutting.

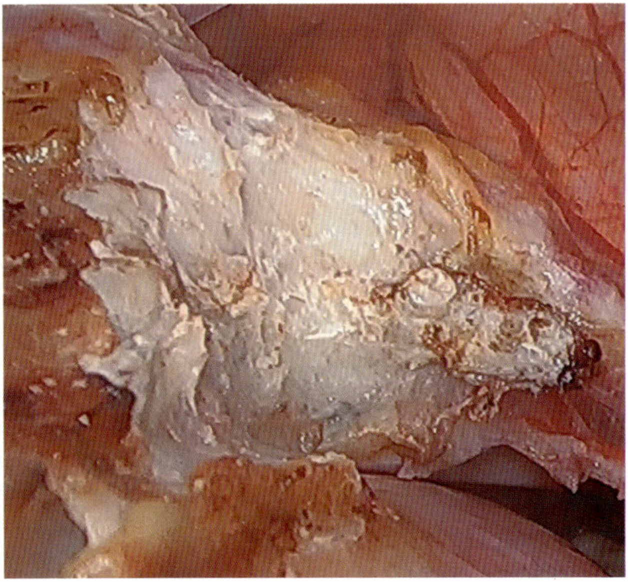

Fig 1.6: Protein denaturation and desiccation in tissue

The effect can be seen in Fig. 1.7.

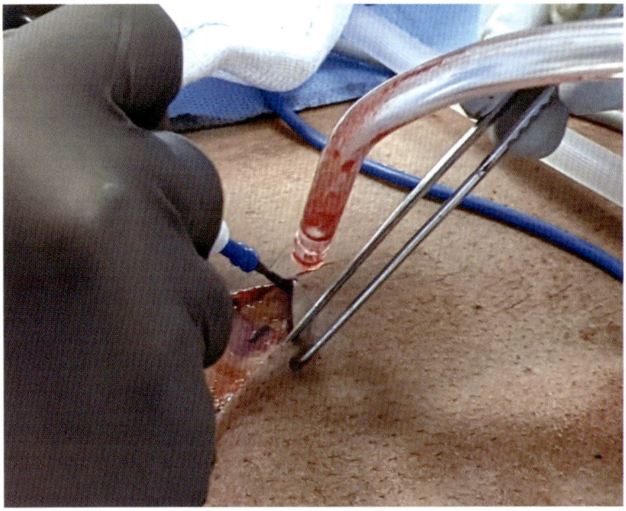

Fig. 1.7: Tissue evaporation causing cut effect

Above 200 degrees, tissue charring starts happening and thus you can see tissue blackening, as can be seen in Fig. 1.8.

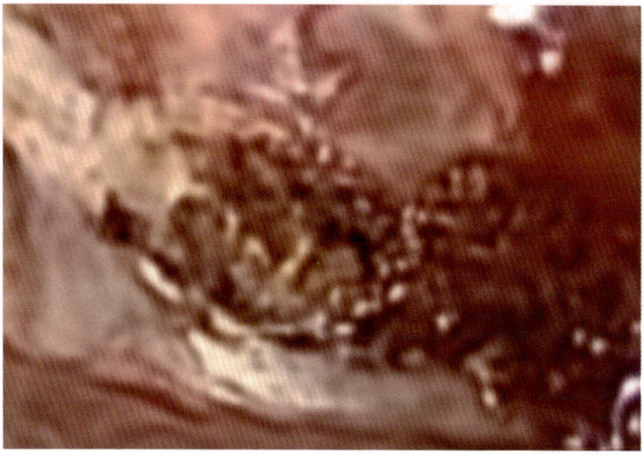

Fig. 1.8: Tissue charring

Factors Affecting Temperature Rise

Temperature rise depends on many factors. Generally, it is a function of:

- **Power setting:** More power setting leads to faster heating of the tissue.
- **Waveform:** This term is defined in the next section. We will see effect of waveform on the tissue in that section.
- **Area of electrode:** Smaller contact area leads to higher concentration of energy and thus higher temperature elevation and *vice versa*.
- **Time duration:** Longer duration of energy delivery leads to higher temperature elevation.
- **Tissue impedence:** Tissue impedance is characteristic of the tissue which opposes flow of current through it. It is function of, among many factors, type of tissue (e.g. fatty tissues have higher impedance compared to regular tissue), water content in tissue (e.g. coagulated tissue has higher impedance).

Understanding Waveforms

Each mode (like Pure Cut, Fulgurate, Precise Bipolar) has a different waveform. Waveform is nature of the current output, which is defined by two characteristics viz. *crest factor* and *impedence response graph*. To understand a mode, it is necessary to understand its underlying charasteristics. Different manufacturers may have different waveforms even though the mode name is the same. Each machine is different and it is useful to understand your electrosurgical unit like your baby. The charasteristics are defined in the following paragraphs.

Crest Factor

Technically, crest factor is defined as ratio of peak voltage to 'average' voltage. Crest factor varies for different modes because not all modes deliver continuous energy. In fact, except pure cut, desiccate and bipolar coagulation modes, all other modes are made up of delivery of energy followed by pause and this pattern is repeated. We do not feel the pauses while using electrosurgical unit because this pattern is repeated at a very fast pace, normally at more than 100 times per second.

To elaborate this, let's take two extreme example viz. one with the lowest crest factor (pure cut) as seen in Fig. 1.9A and one with the highest crest factor (spray coagulation) as seen in Fig. 1.9B. Intuitively, you already know that spray coagulation causes more spark compared to pure cut at the same power setting.

Crest factor has the following implications:

- Higher crest factor leads to more depth of effect. Subsequently, modes with higher crest factors cause more coagulation

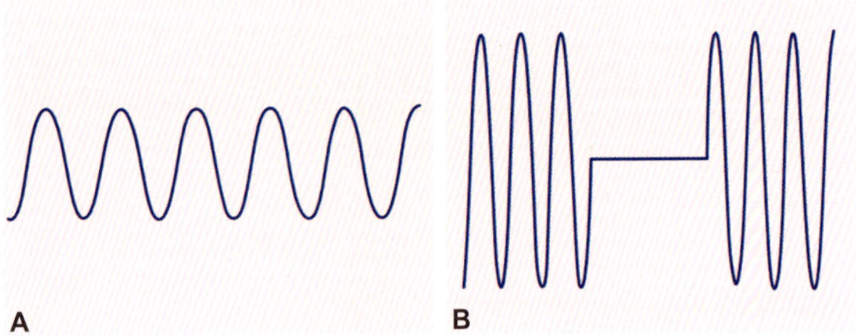

Fig. 1.9: Crest factors for two modes in monopolar (A) Pure cut; (B) Spray coagulation

because they work on larger area, their energy is spread and thus causes lower temperature elevation.

- High crest factor modes can cause spark. Used in the right manner, they can be useful in superficial coagulation.
- While working on vascular tissues, it is better to use modes with moderate crest factor even for cutting. This causes some amount of cutting on the side walls.

Impedance Response Graph

Impedance response graph is the graph that plots actual power delivery by an electrosurgical unit against tissue impedance.

Different manufacturers follow different impedance response graph even though they may use the same name for a mode. Also, within a machine, different modes may have different impedance response graph.

The actual delivery of power is almost always not the same as the set power. The delivered power is typically less than the set power and it is function of tissue impedance and the mode used.

For example, in Fig. 1.10, the impedance response of a machine without tissue sensing is shown, which is 'natural' for

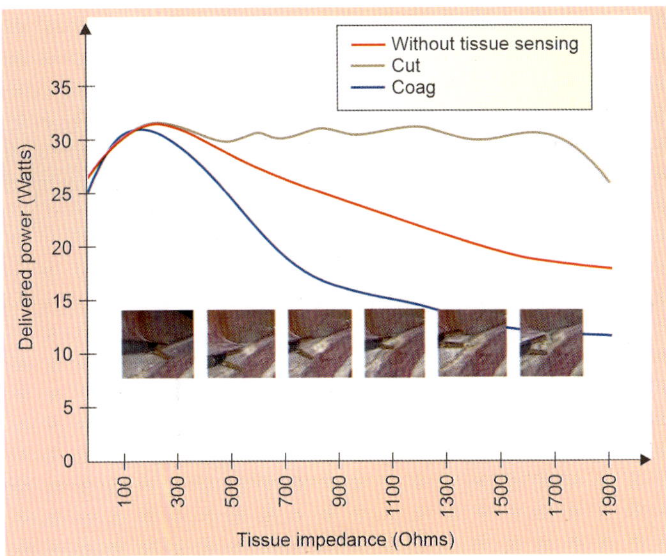

Fig. 1.10: Impedance response graph

a typical circuit. It is beyond the scope of this book to explain the "natural" behaviour of the machine.

Machines with tissue sensing technology can deliver power based on the tissue impedance in such a way that desired tissue effect is achieved. For example, cut current should continue to deliver output at high level (close to set power) even though tissue impedance keeps on increasing as a result of heating of the tissue. That's why the cut impedance response graph stays at higher power even though tissue impedance keeps increasing. Conversely, coagulation impedance response graph reduces the power delivery as a result of increase in tissue impedance. This ensures that the tissue after coagulation, i.e. after reaching 60–80 degrees of temperature and with higher impedance, the power delivery reduces so that the temperature does not rise much beyond that. This ensures a good coagulation, without causing cutting effect or charring.

Thus, machines with tissue sensing technology can deliver smoother cuts and better coagulations.

With the above fundamental concepts, now you are equiped to understand your electrosurgical unit and use it effectively and safely.

The following section describes various tips, which are based on practical experience and understanding of the above concepts.

Safety Hazards and Precautions

The next section on tips covers some of the safety precautions in details. These hazards and the precautions are summarised in the Table 1.2.

Table 1.2: Safety hazards while using electrosurgical units, their causes and preventive measures

Safety hazard	*Cause*	*Precautions*
Patient plate burns Fig. 1.11A	+ Insufficient contact area + Non-suitable area	+ Use disposable plates because they come with adhesives + Use split patient plates and electrosurgical unit that can detect insufficient contact

Contd.

Table 1.2: Safety hazards while using electrosurgical units, their causes and preventive measures *(Contd.)*

Safety hazard	*Cause*	*Precautions*
		+ Avoid areas such as hairy, having scars + Do not wrap wet cloth around the patient plate
Alternate site burns Fig. 1.11B	HF leakage + Current finds alternate path to reach ground Examples + Patient hand touching saline stand that is grounded + Surgeon sitting on a stool that is grounded	+ Insulate the operating area from the ground + Use electrosurgical unit that can detect HF leakage
Remote Tissue Damage Fig. 1.11D	+ Capacitive coupling Example: During gall-bladder surgery, cannula touches bowel + Instrument insulation failures	+ Regular visual inspection of instruments + Be aware of risk of capacitive coupling and ensure instruments do not touch other parts during surgery
Surgery Site Fire Fig. 1.11C	+ Inflammables Example: Spirit used for cleaning. The surgery site is still wet and power delivery is activated	+ Dry the surgery area well before power activation
Adjacent tissue damage	+ Direct coupling Example: + Unintended coupling like retractor touches the artery forcep, which is energised by monopolar electrode + Excessive high power/ high voltage + Two electrosurgical units on one patient	+ Be mindful of the risks of direct coupling + Start with lower settings and then increase, if required + Use only electrosurgical unit on one patient

Tips for Safe and Effective Use of Electrosurgical Unit

This section lists and elaborates useful tips for safe and effective use of electrosurgical unit. Given vastness of the subject, this list should not be considered as an exhaustive resource.

Tips for Buying Electrosurgical Unit

Go for electrosurgical unit that does not compromise on safety features. Ideally, it should have the following safety features:

- **Patient plate contact quality monitoring:** This safety feature is a must, given that patient plate burns are the most common thermal damage. This feature is also known by return electrode monitoring and similar names. If there is no sufficient contact between patient plate and the patient, the electrosurgical unit would indicate it and will not allow delivery of output. For this feature to work, the patient plate should be a split one.

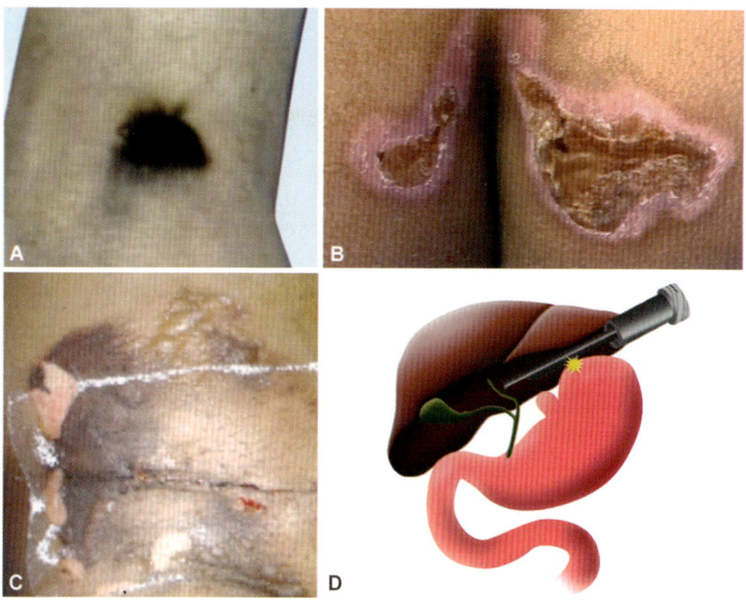

Fig. 1.11: Safety hazards (A) Burns at the site of patient plate; (B) Alternate site burns; (C) Burns due to fire; (D) Remote tissue damage

- **HF leakage monitoring:** During surgery, current may find alternate paths to the ground. There may be burns due to this alternate flow of currents if there is concentration of current at any place in the path. An intelligent electrosurgical unit will detect HF leakage, give alarm and stop delivery of monopolar output.
- **Time-out function:** Electrosurgical unit that has this feature will stop delivery of current if output is activated for a duration more than threshold and also give alarm. This is required to avoid any unintended activation.

The general functionality of electrosurgical unit is also important.

The following are the special cases that are challenging and prove worth of an electrosurgical unit. It is better to evaluate an electrosurgical unit under these conditions (whichever applicable), which clearly differentiate between a good machine and an average machine.

1. **Underwater surgeries:** Underwater surgeries like TUR or surgical hysterescopy are special condition because of very low impdence of the tissue. The ability to provide smooth cut and quick coag in these conditions test performance in low impedance conditions.
2. **Cutting fatty tissues:** Fatty tissues offer high impedance. The ability to provide smooth cut of fatty tissues test performance in high impedance conditions.
3. **Ability to coag in bloody field:** When a bleeder is punctured, a good electrosurgical unit will be able to provide quick control on bleeding.

Other than the above points, it is important to check the following:

1. **General current quality:** Current quality is the ability to cut smoothly, coagulate or seal quickly to avoid much blood loss or smoke, charring.
2. **Multiple cut modes:** A good ESU will have various cut modes in monopolar viz. low, high, pure, blend and endo. These modes are required in specific situations.
3. **Multiple coag modes:** A good electrosurgical unit will have various coag modes (e.g. in monopolar: desiccate, fulgurate, spray and in bipolar: precise, standard and macro).

4. **Intuitive interface:** If the user can start using the machine without demonstration or withour reading user guide, it is a good sign that it is easy to use.[1]
5. **Reliability and service support:** While these factors can be assessed only after purchase, it is a good idea to evaluate the manufacturer on these factors by taking feedback from the existing users.

A Note on Twin Coagulation

There are specific cases, e.g. cardiothoracic surgery or multiple injuries, where two surgeon might be operating on a patient. It is convenient if two surgeons have their respective monopolar pencils.

To support this requirement, ESU manufacturers have developed twin coagulation feature where two monopolar outputs are available from a single ESU. Some manufacturers have implemented it as two simultenous outputs while some manufacturers have implemented it as two alternate outputs (i.e. at a time only one monopolar can be active).

Most of the manufacturers have only one generator inside and the output is split between the two monopolar outputs. As explained in Fig. 1.12, when one of the monopolar outputs is activated, power delivery is as per the settings. However, when both the monopolar outputs are activated, power is divided between them. Existence of two independent generators is proven only if two separate settings for the two monopolars and simultaneous outputs are possible.

Hence, it is recommended that even if you buy an ESU with twin coagulation, the output is used alternatively. There is still a case for buying twin coagulation ESU because having two pencils for two surgeons is a great convenience.

Before Surgery

Understand functionality of the electrosurgical unit: If you are using a particular model for the first time, familiarise yourself with the functionality and safety features of it.

[1]Please note that I am not recommending that user guide should not be read. For getting the best out of the machine, the user guide should be read.

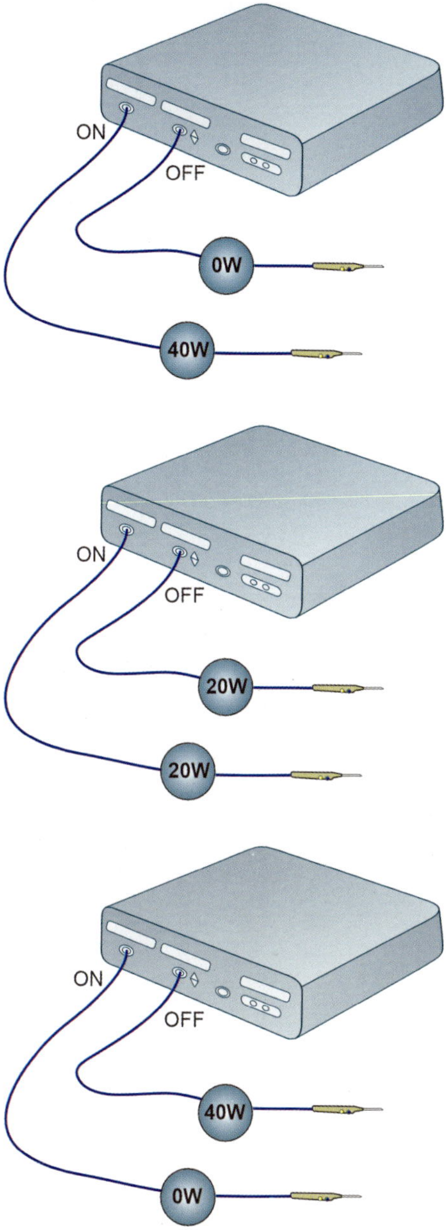

Fig. 1.12: Power delivery in twin output ESUs

Instruments, connectors and cables

- Check for any insulation failures in instruments or cables. If any found, they should be immediately replaced.
- Check that the instruments, cables and the main unit are compatible with each other.
- All cables should be untangled.

Types of patient plates: The safest patient plates are the split disposable types. Split patient plates allow intelligent electrosurgical unit to identify contact quality. Disposable patient plates come with adhesives and hence, contact is maintained even when the patient is moved during surgery. Fig. 1.13 shows a disposable split patient plate.

Split silicon patient plates are the second-best choice and offer cost effective alternative. Fig. 1.14 shows a silicon split patient plate.

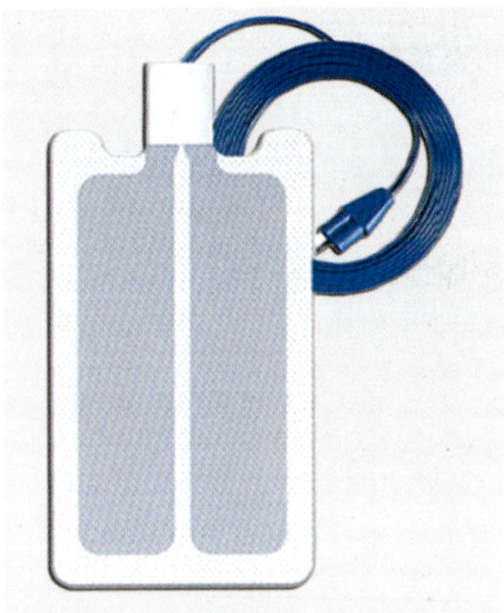

Fig. 1.13: Disposable split patient plate

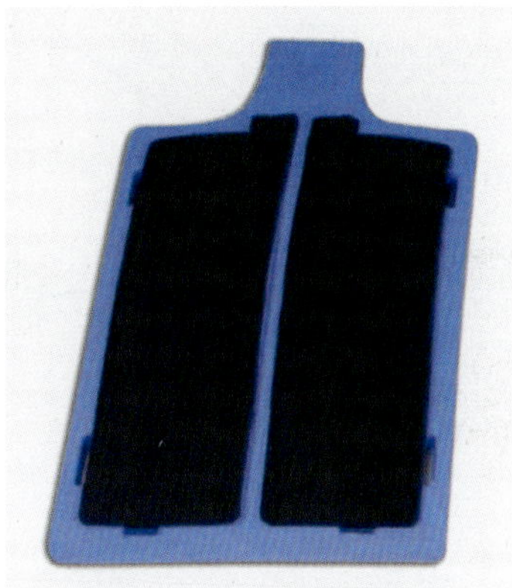

Fig. 1.14: Silicon split patient plate

Disposable and silicon patient plates are available in non-split form as well. Non-split patient plate cannot provide intelligence to the machine about how good the contact is between patient and the patient plate. Hence, they should be avoided. Within these two options, disposable is still a better option due to adhesive which can maintain good contact (Fig. 1.15).

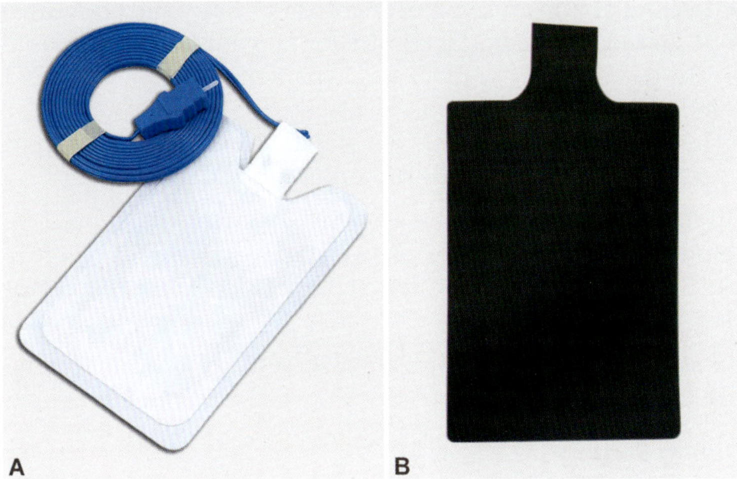

Fig. 1.15: Nonsplit patient plates (A) Disposable; (B) Silicon

Steel patient plates should be avoided because (i) being rigid, provide smaller contact area and (ii) cannot help intelligent electrosurgical unit to assess contact quality.

For silicon patient plates, though not mandatory, applying a conductive jelly will enhance contact quality.

If the patient has pacemaker, consult the pacemaker manufacturer: The older pacemakers may not have filters for the high frequency current generated during electrosurgery. Consult with the pacemaker manufacturer before surgery on the possible impact of high frequency current on the pacemaker.

Just before Surgery

Keep the activation sound volume at audible level: If the sound volume is not audible, any inadvertent activation will not be noticed by you.

Proper placement of patient plate: Patient plate placement plays a key role in safe surgery and also in effective delivery of current while using electrosurgical unit. The patient plate should be placed as per the guidelines below:

- It should be close to the area of surgery but it should not be adjacent as well.

- It should be on muscle area. Avoid fatty, hairy and bony area.
- It should be on a flatter surface for maximising contact area.
- The current path (surgery site to patient plate) should avoid heart, if possible.
- It should be placed in such a way that two parts of (a split) patient plate get roughly same amount of current.

Flammable disinfectants: Flammable disinfectants should be wiped dry and should be allowed to evaporate fully before electrosurgical unit use is started. Otherwise, there is a risk of fire.

Check initial settings: Keep initial power settings to the minimum. Select safe modes.

During Surgery

Start with lower settings, increase if required: The settings should be as low as possible and as high as needed. Power, which is more than required, causes tissue damage and toxic smoke.

Any change in settings should be orally informed by the technician and acknowledged by the surgeon.

Use low voltage waveforms as much as possible: For example, pure cut and desiccate waveforms are lower voltage compared to fulgurate and spray. Higher voltage waveforms cause more spark and may also cause more leakage currents.

Use bipolar than monopolar, wherever possible: Bipolar is a safer mode than monopolar. Thus, wherever possible, bipolar should be preferred.

Do not activate the power when current delivery is not intended: Some surgeons keep the power activated for a long duration even though actual usage is for shorter duration. When the current is not delivered to the tissue, it will likely find alternate paths and can cause unintended damage. Also, higher duty cycle of usage lowers life and reliability of the electrosurgical unit main unit.

If the patient is moved, check the patient plate again: Any movement of the patient body necessitate checking of the patient plate and its proper contact with the patient body.

The active electrode should be visible all the time: The active electrode should preferably be kept in a holster when not in use. In absence of a holster, it should be visible all the time and should not be touching patient body or other conductive items (like metal instruments).

Be attentive to activation and alarm sounds: Advanced surgical diathermies provide distinct activation sounds for different modes (monopolar cut, monopolar coag, bipolar coag). Ensure that the activation sounds are consistent with the expected activated modes.

Also, be attentive for any alarms (visual and audio). Alarm sounds are, as per the standards, at highest volume levels irrespective of volume level set. An advanced electrosurgical unit will give alarms for:

i. Patient plate contact not sufficient,
ii. HF leakage current more than threshold, and
iii. Other errors like bipolar instrument being open (without any continuity) and time-out.

Clean electrodes regularly: Any carbon deposition on electrodes hinder flow of current through the electrode. Hence, electrodes should be cleaned regularly during the surgery. Fig. 1.16 shows (A) electrode with carbon deposition and (B) cleaned electrode.

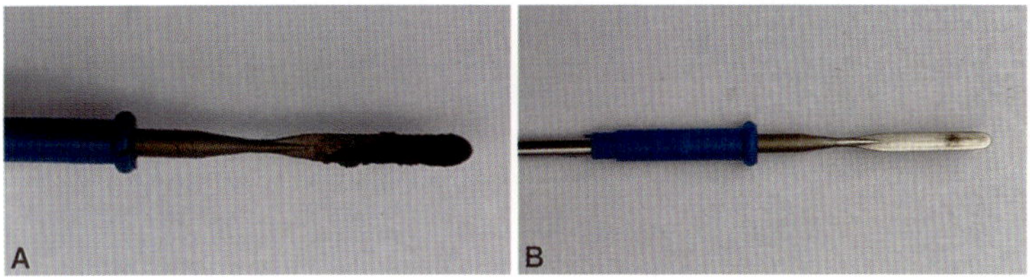

Fig. 1.16: Electrodes (A) Carbon deposition; (B) Cleaned electrode

Avoid tissue sticking to the electrodes: For monopolar open surgery, teflon coated electrodes can be used to reduce tissue sticking. For bipolar, using irrigation by saline can help avoid tissue sticking. Also, in general, clean electrodes cause less tissue sticking.

Keep electrode in your view during activation in a laparoscopic surgery: Activation of power during a laparoscopic surgery should always be done when the camera focuses on the active electrode.

Use all metal or all plastic trocars: Trocars that are combination of plastic and metal for a capacitor and allow for capacitive coupling. This can cause flow of stray current in monopolar mode and cause damage on the abdominal wall.

Ensure the instrument is not touching any other metal parts: Monopolar current may find alternate paths to the patient plate than the surgery site. Such alternate paths should be avoided. The alternate paths are possible due to insulation failures on the instrument or capacitive coupling. Hence, care should be taken that the instruments do not touch any other parts during the surgery.

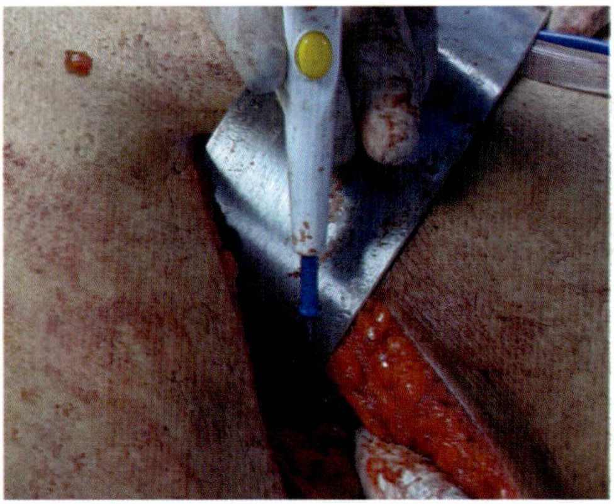

Fig. 1.17: Unintended direct coupling

This is especially important in laparoscopic surgery because the surgeon's vision is limited to the surgery site. In open surgery as well, contact with other metallic instruments (like retractor, as shown in Fig. 1.17) should be avoided.

Be mindful of current density: The increase in temperature depends on the concentration of current. If the current flows through a narrow path of tissues, it can cause thermal enjury there even though the narrow path is away from the surgery site. For example, while cutting an adhesive band between gallbladder and duodenum, if the band is narrower near the duodenum, the current will get concentrated there. It can cause thermal damage to the duodenum which may not be recognised during surgery.

Insulating surgery area from the ground: The surgery set up should be insulated from the ground to avoid HF leakage. Examples are: patient hand touching saline stand, surgeon sitting on a steel stool that does not have bushings on its legs. In both these cases, part of the current flows to the ground through these alternate paths. Surgeons using wooden platform, using non-conductive material for the flooring are some of the solutions.

Evacuate smoke: To reduce effect of toxic gases, use of smoke evacuator or suction machine is recommended during surgery.

After Surgery

Inspect for any thermal damage: Check skin at the patient plate for any thermal damage. Also, inspect the other patient body parts for any thermal damage that can happen due to HF leakage.

Clean instruments and the patient plate: If any jelly is used for silicon patient plate, clean it without rubbing too much. Rubbing the silicon patient plate reduces its conductivity. After cleaning instruments, use of air spray for drying is recommended.

Inspect instruments and cables for any insulation failure: Check for any insulation failures in instruments or cables. If any found, they should be immediately replaced.

Handling of adverse incidents: If any adverse incident has taken place, it should be documented, in as much details as possible, describing nature of incident, sequence of events.

The medical equipments including their settings and instruments should be kept as they are and clinical engineer should be called. Without this, the clinical engineer may not be able to investigate the root cause of adverse incident.

Once the investigation is completed, the learnings should be shared, proactive actions should be taken so as not to repeat the incident.

Basic Troubleshooting

Manufacturers typically provide troubleshooting guide as part of service manual. Many of the troubleshooting procedures are specific to the particular model and it is advisable that either the surgeon, OT technician or biomedical engineer is aware of the trobleshooting procedures.

Flowcharts given in Figs 1.18 and 1.19 are some of the basic troubleshooting procedures for common problems.

Problem: Patient plate error sound and visual indicator

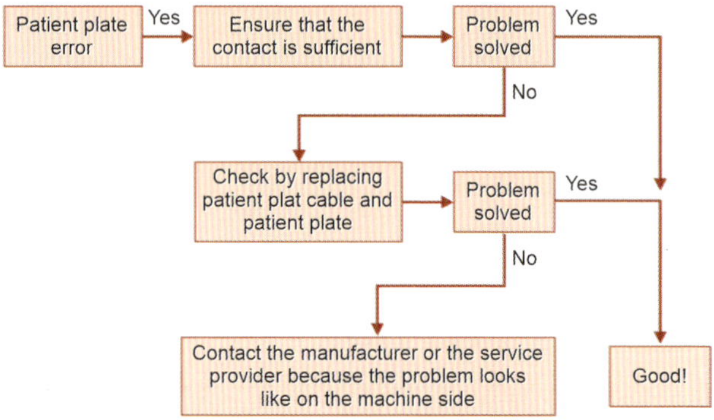

Fig. 1.18: Flowchart for resolving patient plate error and visual indicator

Problem: No power delivery of monopolar even though activation sound beeps

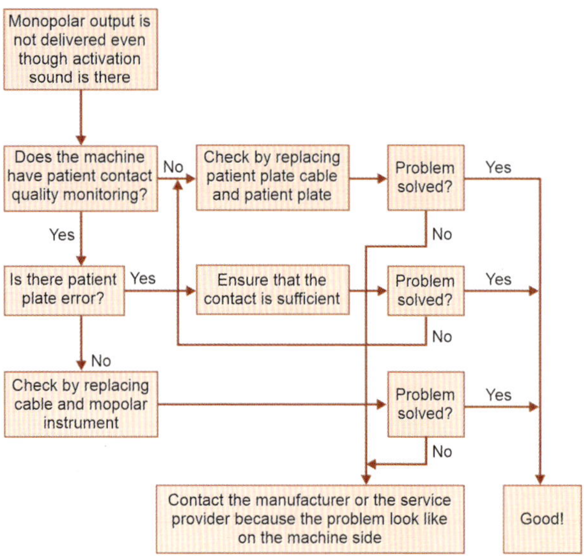

Fig. 1.19: Flowchart for resolving no power delivery of monopolar despite of activation sound

CHAPTER 2

Advanced Energy Sources

Sudarshan Nagaonkar

In this chapter, we will cover advanced energy sources topics viz. ultrasonic scalpel, advanced bipolar (vessel sealer) and saline bipolar.

Ultrasonic Scalpel

Ultrasonic scalpel is a form of mechanical energy (vibrations) that transfer energy to the tissue. The energy creates heat in the tissue and generates cut and coag effects. The instrument also delivers pressure and that is additional form of energy that creates shearing effect.

The ultrasonic scalpel system consists of generator, transducer and hand instrument as shown in Fig. 2.1.

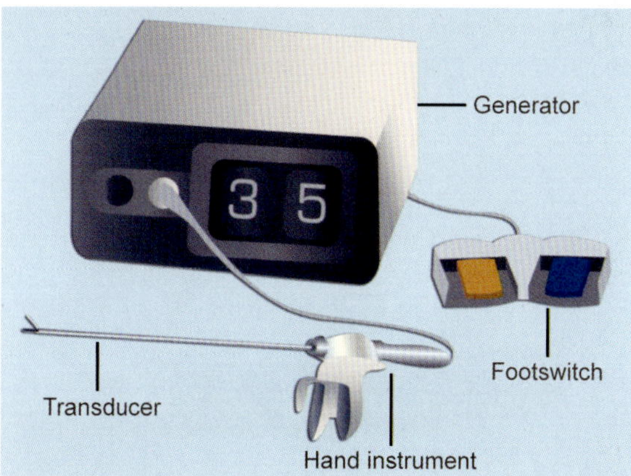

Fig. 2.1: Components of an ultrasonic scalpel system

Generator

The generator delivers electrical energy of ultrasonic frequency (typically 55 kHz) to transducer. The generator also acts as the main user interface for activation, deactivation and controlling power and managing other settings.

Transducer

It converts electrical energy into mechanical vibrations, which are then delivered to the hand instrument.

Hand Instrument

Hand instrument delivers the mechanical vibrations to patient tissue. It is also designed to deliver mechanical pressure in the controlled manner when the mechanical vibrations are delivered to patient tissue.

Working Principle of Ultrasonic Scalpel

The vibrations created are at a frequency (depending on the manufacturer) that is within the range of 23–55 kHz. These are above the range of sound that can be heard by human ear and hence, these frequencies are called as ultrasound. The vibrations are typically longitudinal, as shown in Fig. 2.2 and each excursion is between 50 and 100 μm, depending on the setting.

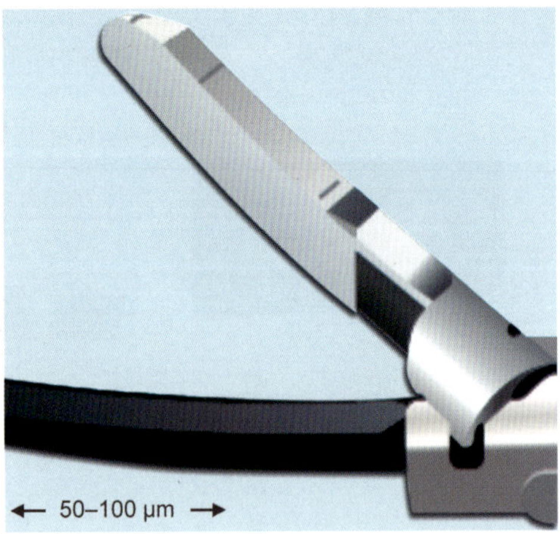

Fig. 2.2: Excursions of an ultrasonic scalpel active blade

The instrument has two blades. Please refer to Fig. 2.3. One blade is oscillating (i.e. carrying the ultrasound energy) and it is non-articulated blade. This blade is also called as active blade. The other blade is non-oscillating (i.e. does not carry ultrasound energy) and it is articulated blade. This blade is called as passive blade.

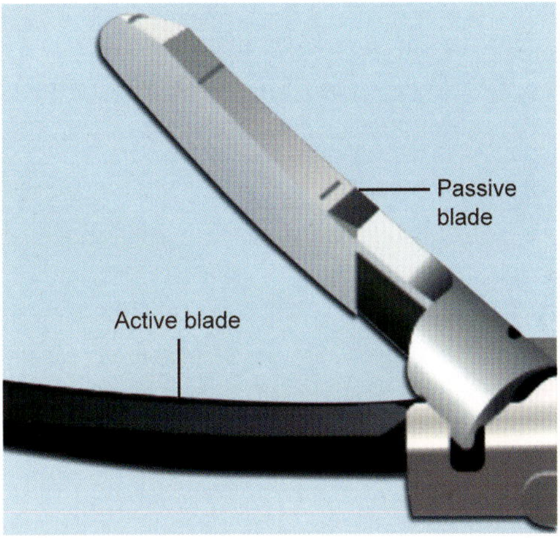

Fig. 2.3: Active blade and passive blade of an ultrasonic scalpel instrument

The ultrasonic energy creates heat in the tissue while the instrument provides compression of the tissue. Depending on the temperature in the tissue, you get different effects like cut and coag.

Due to creation of relative vacuum in the tissue, there is cavitation effect. Cavitation effect is opposite of what we observe in pressure cooker. In the pressure cooker, due to high pressure, the boiling point of water increases. Hence, there is less boiling even after heating so much. The opposite effect (i.e. cavitation effect) is that in low pressures, boiling point of water is lowered. And we know that when water content of cells starts boiling, we get cutting effect. So, in ultrasonic energy system, the cutting effect occurs at lower temperatures than 100 degrees. That's why you see droplets of water instead of vapour when using ultrasonic scalpel. Cavitation effect is a positive aspect of ultrasonic energy because cutting happens at lower temperatures.

The mechanical pressure between the jaw also causes tissue tension and gives strength to the cutting effect.

Application Notes

Understand Factors Affecting Cut and Coag Effects

In ultrasonic scalpel, you will generally get cutting as well as coag effects all the time. Whether cut is dominant or coag, depends on many factors. In the Fig. 2.4, cut is represented by yellow and coag is represented by blue.

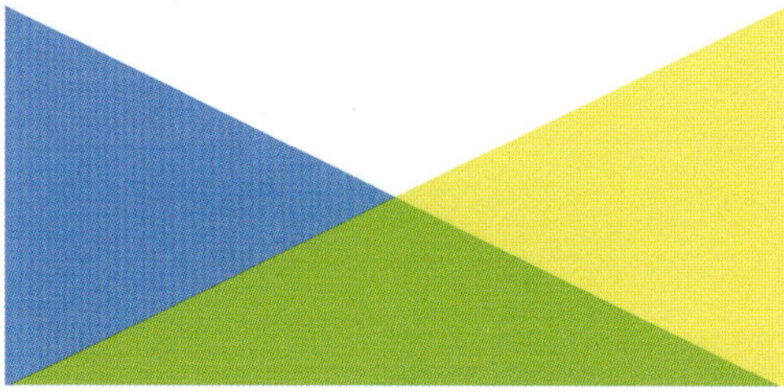

Fig. 2.4: Sprectrum of cut and coag effects while using ultrasonic scalpel

Where exactly on the spectrum the effect will be depends the factors below:

- **Tissue tension:** More tissue tension will cause more cut effect. For example, by lifting the tissue, one can create more tissue tension.
- **Power setting:** Typically, the power setting is Level 1 to Level 5. Higher the power setting, higher will be the cutting effect.
- **Pressure between jaws:** The pressure between the jaw depends on the force applied while closing the jaw and also on the amount of tissue chunk held. Higher pressure will lead to higher cut effect.
- **Jaw sharpness:** If the active jaw is sharp, it will concentrate the energy and have more cut effect. If the jaw is blunt, it will spread the energy and will cause more coag effect.

Using the Active Blade as "Monopolar"

We tend to compare ultrasonic scalpel instrument to bipolar because in the most cases we hold tissue between the jaw. However, unlike a bipolar instrument, it is possible to use only the active blade of ultrasonic scalpel because it carries ultrasonic energy just like you would use monopolar ESU pencil blade.

Understanding Polarity of the Instrument

Bipolar instruments typically have same shape for each of the jaw part. However, ultrasonic scalpel has active blade and passive blade, which differ not only in shape but also that only active blade carries the energy.

When the surgeon is sealing a vessel, it is important to rotate the jaw by 180 degrees and apply energy once again. For example, if you seal a vessel using instrument like in Fig. 2.5A, then delivery energy again using instrument like in Fig. 2.5B. This ensures that both sides of the vessel get adequate energy.

Also, when there are vital organs nearby, it is better to use active blade away from the vital organs.

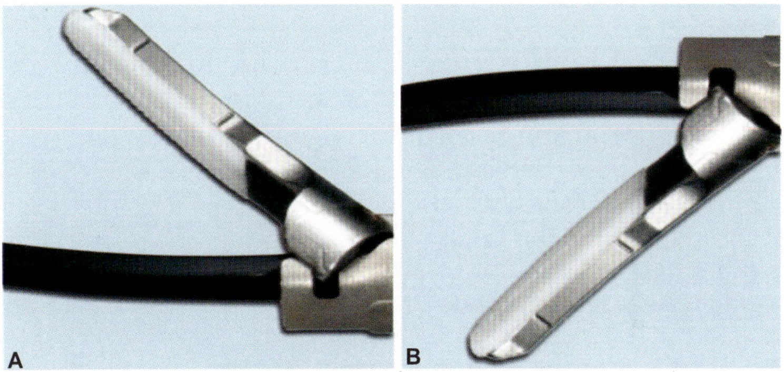

Fig. 2.5: Polarity of energy in ultrasonic scalpel instrument

Safety Precautions

- **The active blade can be hot:** The active blade can reach temperatures of around 200 degrees. It takes upwards of 15 seconds for it to cool down to temperatures that would be acceptable for usage. Particularly, the heated blade should not touch neighbouring vital organs.
- **Avoid premature cutting:** Despite its many advantages, ultrasonic scalpel is not as good for controlling the bleeding. So, ensure that coag is sufficient before cutting is attempted.

Advantages of Ultrasonic Scalpel

Ultrasonic scalpel has many advantages, particularly when compared to electrosurgery.

- A single tool that grasps, dissects, cuts and coagulates
- By using active blade alone, mimic monopolar
  - Single instrument used as 'bipolar' and 'monopolar'
- No tissue sticking
- No smoke or charring
- Less thermal spread
- Better visibility in laparoscopic surgeries
- Safe from most of the thermal injuries
- No interference with implanted devices like pacemaker

Advanced Bipolar (Vessel Sealer)

Advanced bipolar aka vessel sealer is a special type of bipolar that is used for sealing blood vessels reliably. Regular bipolar coagulation cannot seal vessels, particularly large ones, reliably.

The vessel sealer current and the hand instrument work together to fuse vessel walls and create a permanent seal. This combination can also be used for coagulating tissue bundles.

The differences between regular bipolar and vessel sealer is summarised in Table 2.1.

The hand instrument provides optimum pressure, which is required for stopping the blood flow and bringing together the opposite walls of a vessel.

Types of Instruments for Advanced Bipolar

There are many types of instruments available for vessel sealer and they are mainly divided into instrument for open surgery and for laparoscopic surgery.

The following are the ones used in most cases for laparoscopic surgery:

Disposable Instrument that Comes with Blade

The instrument has the following advantages:

- The blade is used for cutting and thus there is no need of separate scissor for cutting and thus change of instrument is avoided.

Table 2.1: Difference between bipolar coagulation and vessel sealer

	Regular bipolar coagulation	*Vessel sealer*
Current continuity	Continuous delivery of current	Algorithmic delivery of current; typically a load of energy for around 0.5 seconds followed by gap of around 0.5 seconds. Many rounds of such energy delivery required until seal is complete.
Wave form	High voltage, low current	Low voltage, high current
Effect	Protein denaturation	Protein denaturation as well as melting of elastin
Thermal spread	More	Less
Tissue fusion	Moderately strong	Strong
Tissue collapse	Moderate	High
Burst pressure	High	Very high

- When cutting happens, the instrument is not moved. This ensures that the cutting is done exactly at the midpoint of the sealed tissue.
- Thermal spread with disposable instrument is lower because only the inner part of the jaw carries current.

The instrument, being disposable, has high recurring cost.

Reusable Instrument with Flat Jaw

The instrument, as shown in Fig. 2.6, is used along with scissor—the instrument is used for sealing a vessel and coagulating tissue bundles and the scissor is used for cutting. This pair is used in two different ways—the instruments are changed through a single port, which adds to the surgery time or the instruments are used through through different ports, which means there is one additional port.

The instrument being a reusable instrument, it reduces recurring cost.

Reusable Instrument with Round Jaw

This instrument, as shown in Fig. 2.7, is getting popular recently. With this instrument, seal and coag is possible with vessel sealer current and cut is also possible with bipolar cut current.

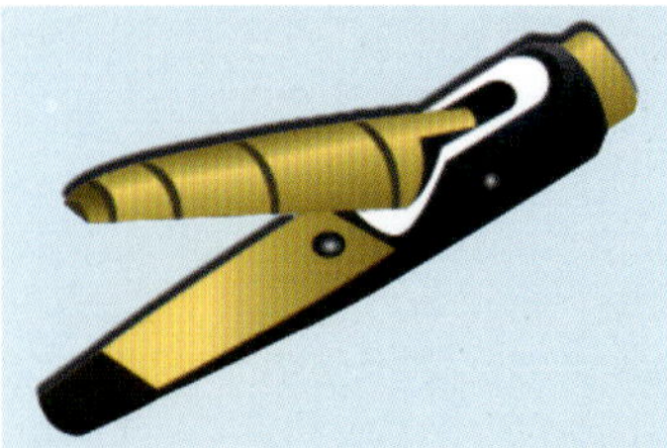

Fig. 2.6: Flat jaw instrument

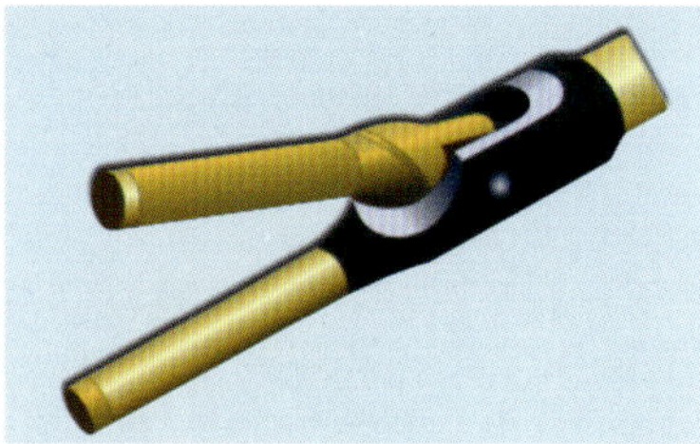

Fig. 2.7: Round jaw instrument

Typically, a large chunk is held between the jaw to seal or coagulate and smaller chunk (and thus higher concentration of current) is held for cutting. Also, holding smaller chunk of ensures that no tissue is cut, which is not fully coagulated. This leads to less bleeding.

Saline Bipolar

Monopolar underwater surgeries like TUR or surgical hysterescopy are done in glycine. Glycine being non-conductive for electric current, monopolar current gets delivered to the tissue near the loop electrode rather than being spread over a large area of tissue.

However, glycine absorbtion in body is toxic and leads to dilutional hyponatremia, also known as TUR syndrome. Longer duration surgeries, leading to higher volume of absorbtion of the irrigant pose higher risk of TUR syndrome.

Studies have shown that with saline as an irrigant, the change in hemoglobin and serum sodium are less compared to glycine. Thus, TUR syndrome is much less likely in the case of saline surgeries.

However, saline being electrically conductive, monopolar does not work. If one uses monopolar in saline, the current will be spread over a large area at the area of surgery and there is hardly any temperature rise. Thus, cutting and coag effects do not occur. This necessitates use of bipolar current, which is known to limit current in small area. The regular bipolar is not effective in highly conductive material like saline and needs a special current.

Saline bipolar current generates heat in the saline solution that causes bubbles. The bubbles get ionised and plasma is formed, which illuminates the loop electrode. Typical plasma around the electrode is shown in Fig. 2.8. The power required to create plasma is high to the tune of 200–300 W. The power required to sustain the plasma is much lower.

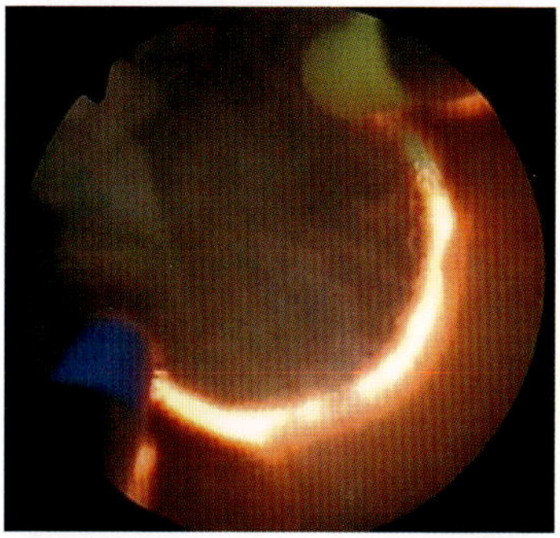

Fig. 2.8: Plasma created by saline bipolar

Saline bipolar current keeps checking the status of plasma and adjusts power on a continuous basis. The power delivered is as low as possible and as high as required to sustain the plasma.

While cutting with plasma, some superficial coagulation happens. Thus, bleeding is less during saline bipolar surgeries.

Laser

Laser is one more energy source that is emerging as a surgeon's choice for certain types of surgeries.

Laser is a special type of light. It does not occur naturally. Einsten theorised first that such a light can be created.

Light is a wave of photons. While laser has all the properties of a light; it has a few special properties:

- **Monochrome:** Laser has a single colour, thus it has a single wavelength.
- **Intense:** Laser has high intensity, thus it carries more energy compared to normal light.
- **Coherent:** Laser waves are not in out of phase with each other. This ensures that their intensity is high.
- **Directional:** Laser does not scatter. That is the reason we use laser pointers and not a torch during our presentations.

Effect of Light on a Material

When any light falls on any material, it can reflect, pass through, scatter or get absorbed. The various movements of light are shown in Fig. 2.9.

Absorption happens when frequency of vibration of electrons in atoms are in tune with frequency of the light. Thus, absorption is selective and also it is material-wavelength combination specific. If the absorption coefficient is higher, the depth of effect is lower and *vice versa*.

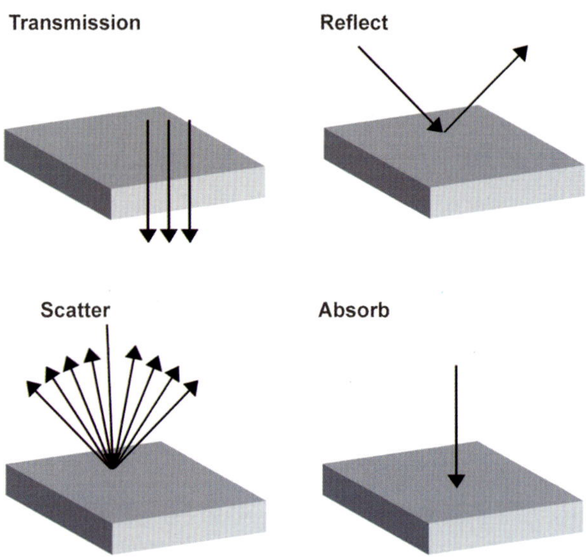

Fig. 2.9: Movements of light

For example, Fig. 2.10 shows absorption coefficient of water and haemoglobin across the wavelengths. It can be seen that water molecules absorb 1470 nm wavelength much higher than 980 nm while hemoglobin absorbs 980 nm more than 1470 nm.

There are no changes in material if the light is reflected, scattered or passes through. However, when light gets absorbed, it can cause changes in the material.

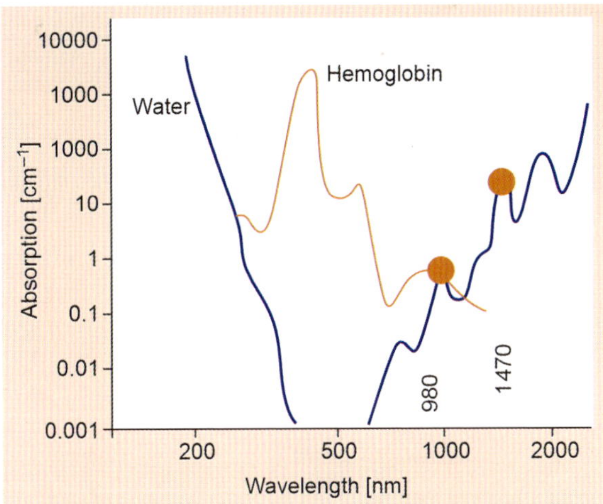

Fig. 2.10: Absorption coefficient of water and hemoglobin across the wavelengths

Most common change in material is generation of heat, photothermal effect. There are also other changes that are possible like:

- **Photomechanical:** Light can cause breaking the bonds in solid materials.
- **Photoacoustic:** Light can generate sound.
- **Photochemical:** Light can cause chemical reaction.

All these effects are wavelength and material dependent. Even if one is changed, the effect may alter or cease completely.

To reiterate, the most common effect is the photothermal effect. This effect is utilised for proctology and varicose vein surgeries.

As we saw in the electrosurgery section, any rise in temperature of tissue has corresponding changes in the tissue. Refer to Table 1.1 (Chapter 1) for convenience.

The rise in temperature is determined by the following factors:

1. Power settings
2. Beam shape
3. Waveform
4. Time duration
5. Absorption coefficient
6. Speed of movement

Types of Fiber

Beam shape of laser beam is decided by the type of fiber used. There are three types of fibers used.

Bare fiber, as shown in Fig. 2.11A delivers energy in concentrated form in the longitudunal direction.

Conical fiber, as shown in Fig. 2.11B delivers energy in a spread manner.

Radial fiber, as shown in Fig. 2.11C delivers energy on the circumference.

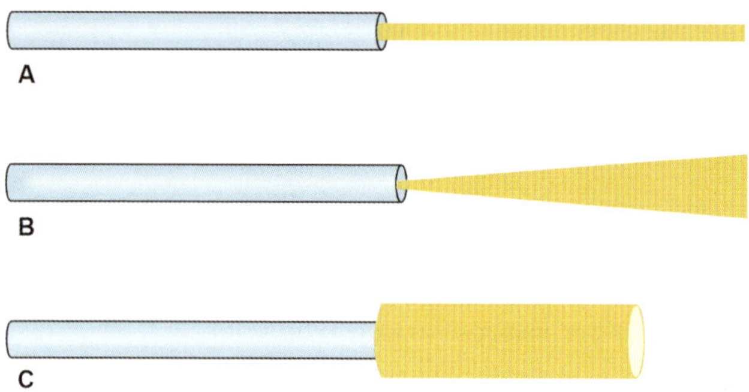

Fig. 2.11: (A) Bare fiber; (B) Conical fiber; (C) Radial fiber

Normally, bare fiber works well for cutting because it causes concentration of energy and thus higher temperature elevation. Bare fiber can also be used for coagulation or ablation when the energy is controlled in such a way that the temperature rise does not go beyond 80 degrees. This can be achieved by stopping the delivery or moving to another tissue that has lower temperature.

Conical fiber is more useful for delivering energy to a larger mass like piles.

Radial fiber is more useful when energy needs to be delivered to the inner circumference of a tunnel like fistula or veins.

Power Energy Equation

Power is rate of energy delivery. Alternatively, energy is power multiplied by time.

$$\text{Energy (joules)} = \text{Power (watts)} \times \text{Time (seconds)}$$

For example, if power of 10 watts is delivered for 5 seconds, the energy delivered will be 50 joules.

A surgeon may decide to deliver 150 joules energy to a pile mass. So, (s)he may set power at 6 watts and deliver energy in 25 seconds.

Specific heat of water is 4.2 joules/ml-degree. It means it takes 4.2 joules of energy to increase the temperature of 1 ml of water by 1 degree centigrade.

Let's take a case of 7 watts power that is delivered to a pile mass having 2 ml of water for 30 seconds. Let's assume that the entire energy is absorbed by the water.

The energy delivered is 7×30 i.e. 210 joules.

The temperature rise in the pile mass is $210/(4.2 \times 2)$, i.e. 25 degrees. So, if the starting temperature of the pile mass was 37 degrees, it will reach 62 degrees.

Since there is a need to limit the energy delivered to the tissue, the laser units have timer function, which stops the delivery after expiry of the timer. For example, you may set 12 watts power and deliver it for 10 seconds for a 1 cm length of a fistula track.

Waveforms in Laser

Lasers can deliver a continuous wave or in a high frequency pulse.

A continuous waveform, as shown in Fig. 2.12A, delivers peak set power all the time.

A pulsed waveform, as shown in Fig. 2.12B, delivers peak set power for certain duration (called as T_{on}) and delivers zero power for certain duration (called as T_{off}). This cycle is repeated.

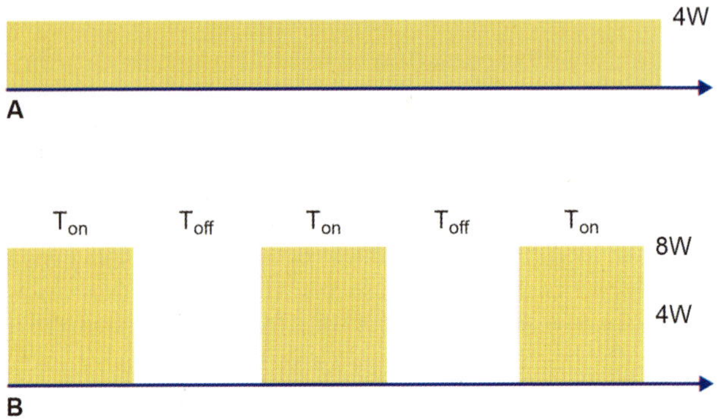

Fig. 2.12: (A) Continuous wave; (B) Pulsed mode

So, the effective power is

$$\text{Peak power} \times (T_{on} / T_{on} + T_{off}).$$

For example, if the peak power is at 8.0 watts, T_{on} is 400 ms T_{off} is 100 ms, then the effective power will be 6.4 watts.

The pulsed waveform achieves the following:

- Increases depth of the effect without increasing the total power.
- Allows the tissue to "relax", i.e. dissipate the heat to the neighbouring tissues.

Pulsed mode is useful when we need to deliver energy to a larger area.

Safety Precautions for Lasers

All the persons inside the OT should wear safety googles when laser is fired. Even after wearing safety googles, it is not advisable to direct laser into eyes.

Laser can reflect from the shiny instruments. It is better to use instruments that come with less reflective coating

CHAPTER

3

Medical Lighting

Sudarshan Nagaonkar

The main intention of the medical lighting is to show tissue in its actual colour to the surgeon. It could be OT light for an open surgery, light source during laparoscopic surgery or spot light during diagnostic examination. We will cover the light as well as movement of the light source in this chapter. Mastery of this topic will help you select the right medical lighting product and utilise it in more effective manner.

In this, chapter, we will cover the fundamentals of this technology, get you familiar with the terms used commonly related to this technology, discuss the do's and don'ts and some basic troubleshooting techniques.

Fundamentals of Light

A white light contains all the rainbow colours. Different colours of light have different wavelength. Our eyes are trained to see in the most natural way for sunlight. Specifically, the noon sunlight is the best light for our eyes to see the real colours. The noon sunlight has all the colours present in it in certain proportions, as shown in Fig. 3.1.

When light falls on an object, which is of, say blue colour, all the other lights than blue get absorbed by the object and the blue light is reflected from it. The reflected light is sensed by our eyes and thus we recognise that object as blue. That is why composition of a light plays important part in the ability to show true colours of any object.

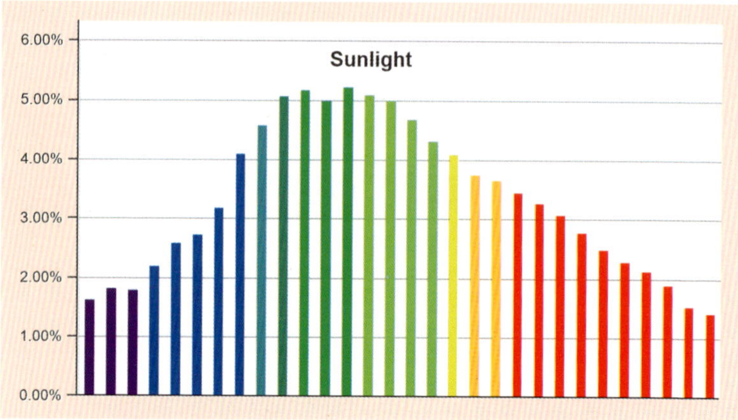

Fig. 3.1: Sunlight composition in 10 nm bandwidths

Technologies for Generation of Light

There are broadly three technologies for light generation viz. LED, halogen and xenon. While halogen light is slightly yellow light, xenon light is slightly blue light.

LED lights have typical life of 50,000 hours while halogen (500 hours) and xenon (1000 hours) have much lower life.

Also, it is important to note that LED lights technology has advanced recently and has overcome its earlier limitations. Specifically, the following advancements are particularly important:

1. Colour stabilisation: LED lights of a few years ago did not have stabilised colour. So, it was possible that two LED lights from same manufacturer varied the colour slightly. With recent developments, the LED lights have colour stabilisation that works with accuracy of ±2% over many years.
2. Higher luminance per wattage: The efficiency of LED lights is much better than halogen and xenon lights. The good news is that the efficiency continues to improve. The side effect of this development is that the heat generated by LED lights is getting lower and lower.

tAlong with composition of light, a light has other characteristics like colour temperature and colour rendering index.

The next section which describes medical grade light, cover these terms and more.

Medical Grade Lights

Medical grade lights are the lights that are fit to use in medical context. Here are four important characteristics of medical grade lights:

Colour Temperature

Technically speaking, it is temperature at which a black body would emit radiation of the same colour as a given object. Colour temperature is conventionally expressed in Kelvins, using the symbol K. As seen in the Fig. 3.2, the colour temperature of around 5500 K is closer to the noon Sunlight. This is the whitest colour, which helps us to identify the true colours of the objects under this light.

It is recommended that lights selected have the colour temperature of around 5500 K.

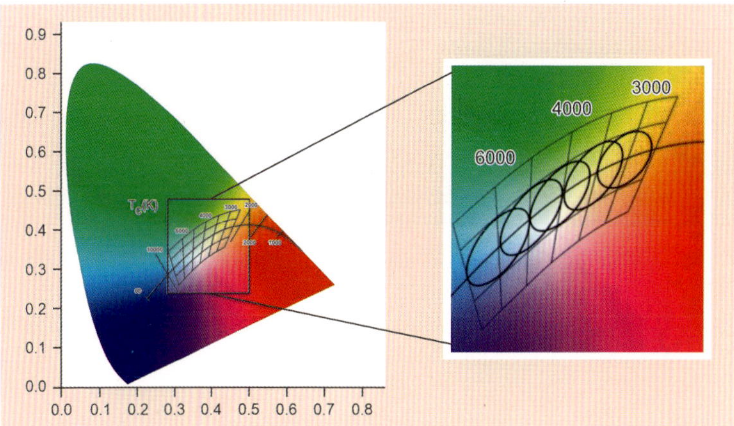

Fig. 3.2: Colour of light at different colour temperatures

Colour Rendering Index

Colour rendering index is a quantitative measure of the ability of a light source to reveal the colours of various objects faithfully in comparison with an ideal or natural light source.

The requirement of a good light (from the correct perceived colour point of view) are:

1. displays a vast variety of colours
2. makes it easy to distinguish slight shades of colour, and
3. the colours of the objects look natural

Colour rendering index is designed to measure the ability of the light source to achieve the above objectives. It is a quantitative measure whose maximum value can be 100, which the most ideal light.

A light having all the colours (rainbow colours) in right proportion will have high colour rendering index. Spectral distribution of warm LED light and cool LED light is shown in Fig. 3.3 as against the spectral distribution of sunlight. Since their spectral distributions are not the same as sunlight, their colour rendering indices are not 100.

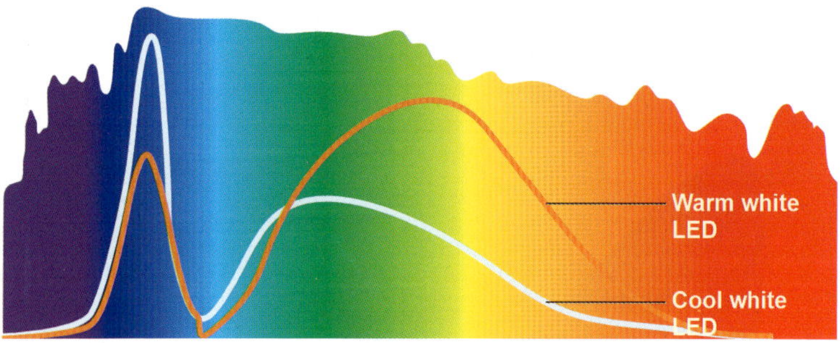

Fig. 3.3: Spectral distribution of sunlight vs LED lights

Medical grade light will have colour rendering index more than 90.

Stable Colour Temperature across Intensities and over Long Life

While colour temperature is important, it is also important to maintain the stable colour temperature across intensities. Medical grade lights will maintain the same colour temperature even at lower intensities such as 2% or 5%. The colour temperature is also maintained by them even after many years of usage.

Truncated Light (Absence of Ultraviolet and Infrared Lights)

The visible light ranges from R (red) to V (violet) in VIBGYOR. Any light below the visible frequency range is called as infrared and any light above the visible frequency range is called ultraviolet light. It is well known that the invisible lights are harmful to the human body (particularly skin and hair). While it may acceptable for a patient to be exposed to such a light once, repeated exposure to the surgeon and the staff is not advisable. So, the surgeons should look for lights that have nil invisible lights. Medical grade lights ensure that this requirement is also met.

Operational Considerations for Light

Shadow-less Light

The fundamental property of light is to travel in straight line and thus cause shadows. While it is not possible to change property of light, it is possible to arrange light in such a way that shadow is minimised. So, please understand that shadow-less is just a marketing word and the actual meaning it less-shadow.

Compare shadow of a cricket player in a day match to the shadow in a night match. In the first case, the shadow is thicker while in the second case there are multiple weak shadows. This happens because in the second case, there are multiple light sources. The same principle is used in operation theatre lights.

Different manufacturers achieve shadow-less performance differently. Therefore, it is recommended that you check the shadow-less performance by obstructing the light with your head or hand closer to the light.

Smoothness of the Movement and Stability

When the surgeon is moving the OT light to illuminate the surgery area, his/her focus is on the surgery area. The movement should be so smooth that without looking at the dome, he/she is able to adjust the light in a smooth and easy manner. Also, once the surgeon releases the dome, it should remain stable at exactly the same position that was released.

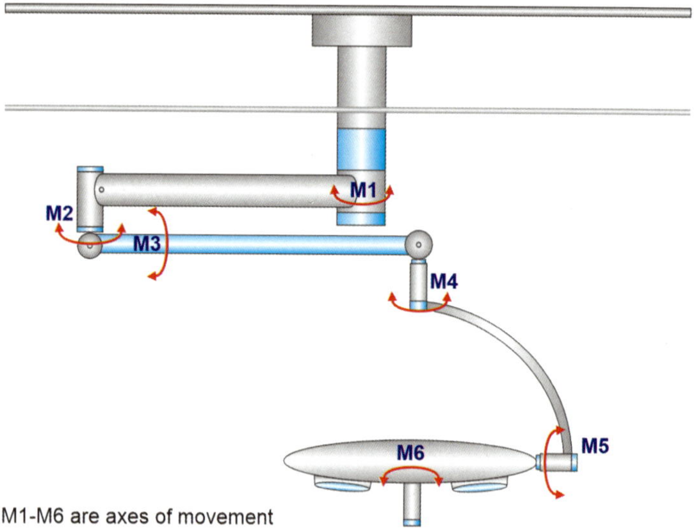

Fig. 3.4: Rotational movements available in a good OT light

More the number of axes of movement, easier it is for the surgeon or the assistant to move the dome. For example, OT light in Fig. 3.4 comes with 6 axes of movements and they are easy to handle compared to the lights that come with just, for example, 3 movements.

360° Motions

The motions of the light dome should be 360° without any stopper. This ensures the movement is without any restrictions and is achieved in less time.

Focus of Light

When the light is fully focused, the radius of the light should be at least 15 cm or 6 inch. This is the minimum amount of area that needs light during surgery. When the light is gradually defocused, it should increase its radius up to 30 cm or 12 inch gradually while maintaining the circular shape and uniformity of light intensity. Beyond this radius, it does not matter if it maintains the circular shape or uniformity of light intensity anyway because the resultant intensity (because of spreading the light) would be lower than practically required for surgery.

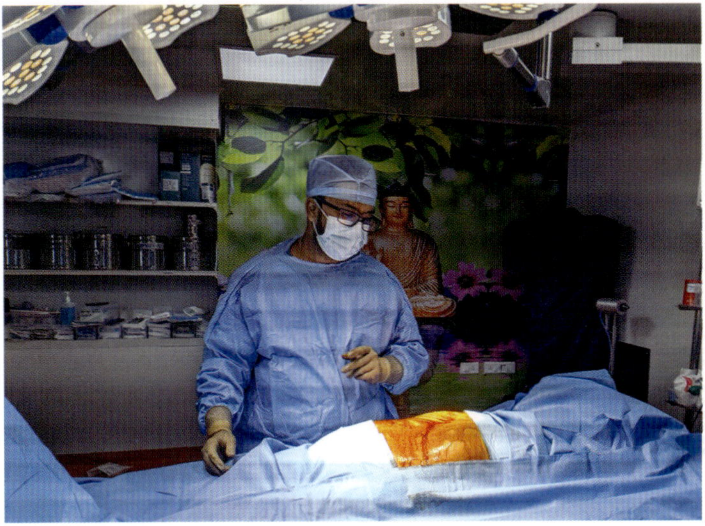

Fig. 3.5: Operational distances in OT light set-up

Typically, the distance between the light and the surgery area is 100 cm. The typical distances are given in Fig. 3.5. However, the focus of the light should be achievable at distance of at least 70 cm and up to 120 cm because it is not possible, in many cases, to maintain the exact distance of 100 cm.

Intensity of Light

Generally, it is accepted that intensity of around 60,000 lux is sufficient for most applications. It should be possible to vary intensity in granular steps (e.g. 1% per step) so that you can set the intensity at the desired level. Some applications like laparoscopic surgery need light at around 5,000 lux to provide ambient lighting. So, it should be possible to set low percentage of intensity.

Lux meter can be used by you to check if the light is giving the promised intensity.

Heat Generation

The LED lights do not elevate the operating area temperature as much as halogen and xenon. Look for LED lights that limit the heat generation to elevation of up to 4 degrees, preferably within 2 degrees.

Suitability for Laminar Flow System

The OT light dome should not obstruct the laminar air flow. So, the domes should be aerodynamic and in petal shape.

Selecting the Right Configuration

Number of Domes

Different applications need different number of domes. Typically, surgeries done at multiple sites would need more number of domes. The most commonly followed convention is given in Table 3.1.

Table 3.1: Selecting number of domes based on application

Number of domes	*Applications*
One dome	Day care surgeries, minor surgeries.
Two domes	Surgeries with large operative area or more depth requirement.
Three domes	Cardio-thoracic, trauma (multiple injury), where two surgeons may operate on a single patient

Light Intensity

Different manufacturers and within a manufacturer, different models have different peak intensity.

The following factors should be considered for deciding peak intensity requirements:

- **Depth of operative area:** The required intensity is dependent upon the depth of the operative area from the surface. For example, skin or hair surgeries would not need more than 50000 lux, while gynaecology surgeries may require 80,000 lux or more.

- **Size of operative area:** If your operative area is bigger in size, you may prefer higher intensities so that even slight defocused light would give you wider area and still maintain the required intensity level.

Ceiling or Wall-mounted or Mobile

You have the choice of going for ceiling or wall mounted or mobile options.

- **Ceiling:** If surgeon's operative room is fixed, ceiling light is most ideal. As it gives the flexibility of movement without any obstructions like mobile light which comes in way while moving within OT.
- **Wall mounted:** This option is rare but used in certain cases where ceiling is too low. This limits the movement within the operating room and hence this option is used only if the ceiling option is not feasible.
- **Mobile or portable:** The advantage of mobile or portable light is its own movement, which allows it to be moved from one room to other room, or sometimes temporarily converting a single surgeons OT to two surgeons OT.

Practical Tips on Effective Use of Medical Lighting

Before Surgery

Ensure that there are no obstacles in the expected path of domes. The obstacles could be pendants, tall stands or trolleys. This ensures that collissions do not occur during the surgery when the staff is more focused on getting the dome position right.

Check to ensure that the movement is neither too tight nor too loose. The movement can be corrected by biomedical engineer or your OT staff provided they have been given training during the installation about corrections.

Most domes have the settings panel on them on one side of the dome. The dome should be rotated in such a way that the settings panel faces the outer side. This helps the circulating staff to change any settings without violating the sterile zone.

During Surgery

It is important to set the right intesity of light. Less intensity reduces quality of vision. Higher intensity than required reflects more causing glare, causes more heat and causes more dispersement.

The focus control decides the diameter of the light at a particular horizontal plane. Typically, the light spread is as per given in Fig. 3.6.

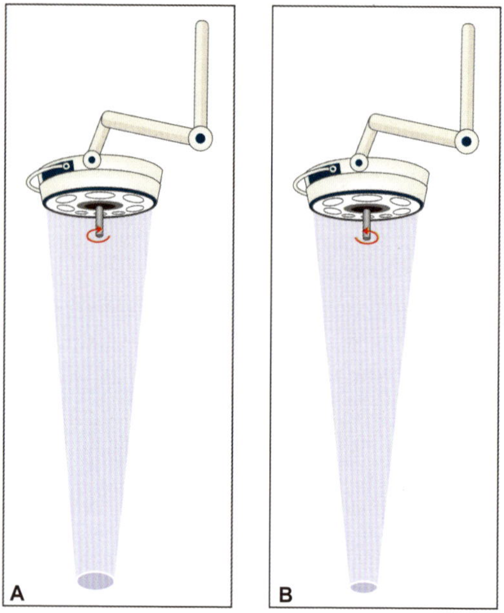

Fig. 3.6: Focus control of an OT light
(A) Bigger radius focus; (B) Small radius focus

Having the right focus that includes the surgery site and excludes the non surgery site helps in concentration of light and thus focus of the mind.

After Surgery

Cleaning of the handle and dome is recommended after surgery. Typically, handles are sterlisable and if the handle has been touched by the sterile team member, it is recommended to clean the handle with care and sterlise it post surgery.

CHAPTER 4

Medical Optics

Sudarshan Nagaonkar

Optical systems have wide usage including laparoscopy, endoscopy, microscopy. This chapter will cover mainly laparoscopic camera system. We will be covering the elements in the system, some key terminologies and the factors that decide quality of image.

The camera system works in parallel to how human vision system works. We see an object only when light falls on it and reflects from it. The reflected light falls on retina through pupil. Retina sends the sensed image to the brain. Until the brain processes the image, it cannot receive any further information from retina. Our eyes can move in upward/downward or sideways. Because of two eyes receiving visual information from slightly different angles, we can understand the depth and have 3D perception.

Basics of Video

Let us get familiar with the basic terms and the technology first.

A video, as demonstrated in Fig. 4.1, is nothing but a series of pictures played at a fast speed. A picture (also called as frame) is matrix of pixels.

Pixel

In digital formats, every image is a collection of "dots". Each "dot" carries a colour and when they are arranged together we get an image.

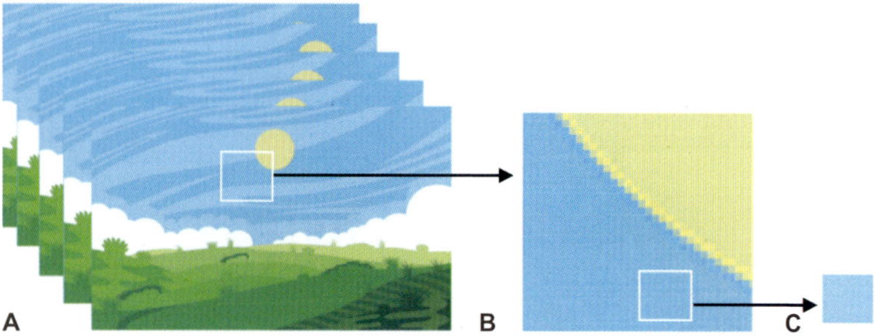

Fig. 4.1: Construction of a video (A) Number of frames; (B) A frame; (C) Pixels within a frame

Thus, pixel is the smallest element in an image and a pixel will have only one colour at a time.

For example, an icon for pencil looks as  but when it is zoomed, it looks as shown in Fig. 4.2.

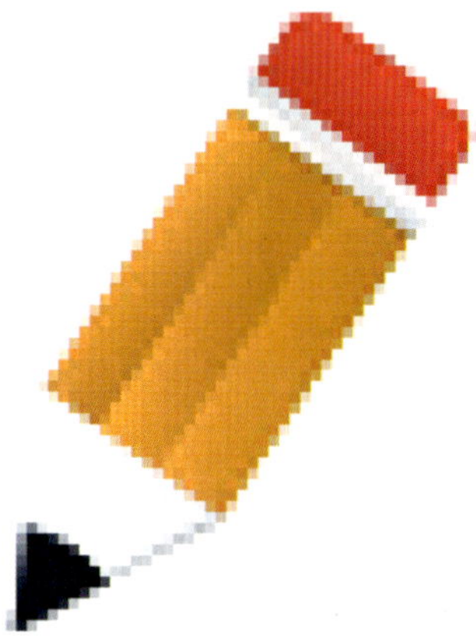

Fig. 4.2: An image made up of pixels

Each of those small squares is a pixel.

Since the pixels are tightly packed in an image and the pixels are so tiny, we see the full image and not any specific pixels.

If the physical size of the pixel is less than 8 microns, a normal human eye cannot see the specific pixel but can see the full image.

Colour or Pixel Depth

Every colour can be represented as a combination of 3 primary colours viz. red, green and blue. For example, yellow is 50% red and 50% green. Number of colours per pixel refers to the number of possible colours that any pixel can represent. While theoretically, infinite number of colours are possible, any digital system can handle a finite number of colours. High number of colours show gradients in more natural way and show colours more truthfully. The gradient is more smooth in Fig. 4.3B compared to Fig. 4.3A because the pixel depth is higher.

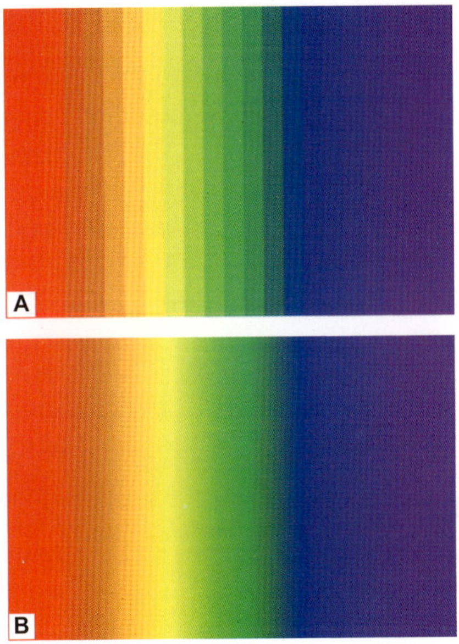

Fig. 4.3: A spectrum of colours (A) When the pixel depth is lower; (B) When the pixel depth is higher

Image Size or Frame Size

Image size or frame size is normally measured as number of columns and number of rows of pixels in an image.

Various image sizes prevalent are given in Table 4.1.

Please note that the frame size is not standardised and the above sizes are only indicative. It is always better to enquire

Table 4.1: Frame sizes in various formats

Format	*SD*	*HD*	*Full-HD*	*4K*
Format name	Standard definition	High definition	High definition /2K	Ultra high definition
Frame size in pixels x pixels	720 × 576	1280 × 720	1920 × 1080	3840 × 2160
Frame size in mega-pixel	0.41	0.92	2.07	8.29
Aspect ratio	Currently 16:9. Earlier 4:3.	16:9	16:9	16:9

exact pixel × pixel size. For example, SD for some people may mean 640 × 480 while for some people it may mean 720 × 576.

Aspect ratio is the ratio of width to height in an image. Earlier 4:3 aspect ratio was the most common. These days, 16:9 aspect ratio is the most common.

Higher the image size, more granular details are available.

Frame Rate

Frame rate is the rate at which the images are captured and played back on the monitor. The most common frame rate is 50 Hz. It means 50 images are captured per second and played on the monitor. The human brain cannot process more than 50 frames per second. Since the images change rapidly, we do not notice individual images but we get feel of a continuous video. In general, for surgery, frame rate does not matter as much as the quality in each frame.

Signal to Noise Ratio

Signal to Noise ratio signifies the ability of the camera to filter out impurities during the image sensing.

Noise is any unwanted or impure information while signal is the physical landscape that we want to capture using the camera. High quality sensors have better ability to accept the physical landscape while filtering out any unwanted information. High quality sensors thus capture image that is closer to the physical objects.

Light Sensitivity

Each camera sensor has certain light requirements to provide acceptable image quality. The best sensors work with lower light requirement and thus do not compromise image quality even in low intensity of light.

Dynamic Range

Dynamic range is the range between two points in a single frame, where the first point is the lowest bright point and the second point is the highest bright point, in such a way that both the points are captured to the satisfaction of the viewer.

Dynamic range is a property of the whole optical system including camera sensor, which is a primary source of this property.

Zoom (Optical and Digital)

When the zoom function is used, it brings a smaller area into the purview of the user. This zoom can be achieved by optical methods. When optical method is used, it uses lenses to spread the incoming light. So, this zoom is achieved mostly without any image degradation. Optical zoom happens before image sensor.

Digital zoom is achieved by processing the parts of the image and magnifying those using software. Digital zoom happens after image sensor. Since this is a lossy function (meaning it causes loss in image quality), manufacturers allow digital zoom only up to a level, so that degradation is not so much.

System Components

Light Source

Light source determines the intensity and quality of light that falls on the tissue. Light source is characterised by type of technology (halogen, xenon, LED), light intensity, colour temperature, colour rendering index. The light source have been discussed in details in Chapter 3: Medical Lighting, for generation of light section.

Fiber Optic Cable

The cable carries light from the light source till the telescope. A fiber optic cable contains thousands of fibers, each fiber of 20–150 microns in diameter. While light travels in vacuum in a straight line, the fiber cables ensures that the light effectively travels in longitudanal direction of the fibers, due to internal reflection, even though the fibers do not form a straight line.

Telescope

Telescope not only carries light from the fiber optic cable but also carries the reflected light from the surgical field to the camera head.

Telescopes come in different sizes and are denoted by the diameter. The typical sizes are 5 mm and 10 mm. Other sizes are 4 mm and 12 mm in diameter.

Telescopes are also characterised by the optical axis. Optical axis is the angle between the central focus of the telescope and the direction of the telescope. For example, in Fig. 4.4A, the telescope is 0 degree and in Fig. 4.4B, the telescope is 30 degrees.

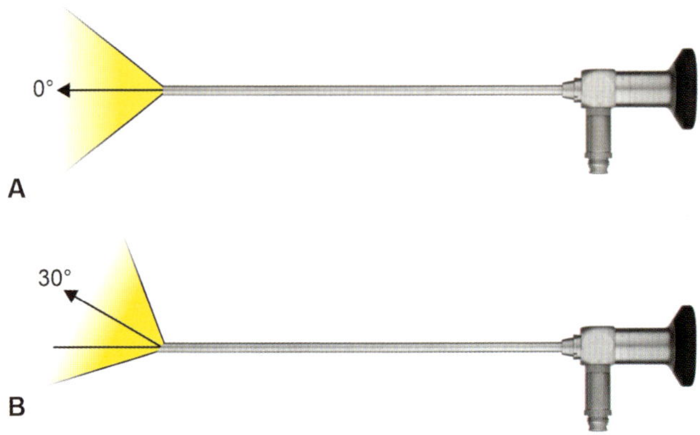

Fig. 4.4: (A) 0-degree telescope; (B) 30-degrees telescope

The most common optical axes are 0 degree and 30 degrees. For special applications, telescopes with 45 degrees or even 120 degrees optical axis are also available.

The other important characteristic of a telescope is the number of rod lenses. The Fig. 4.5 shows the construction of telescope. Rod lenses play a major role in deciding quality of a telescope.

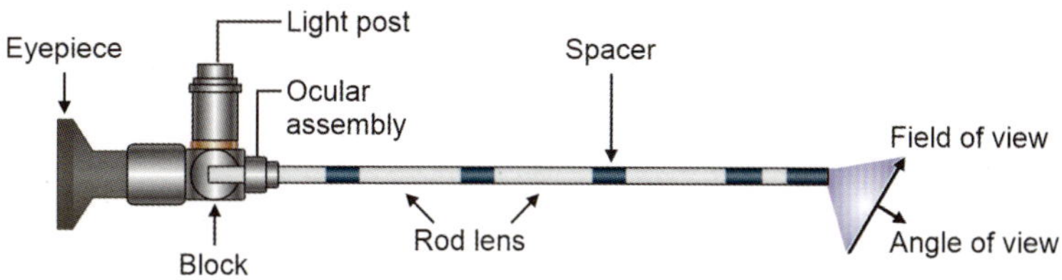

Fig. 4.5: Construction of telescope

Rod lenses are made up of glass. Rod lenses are coated to avoid light reflecting from the road lense surface. Higher number of rod lenses mean less air gaps within the telescope, leading to better image quality.

Rod lenses which have materials with high transparency and better coating, provide better image quality.

Camera Head

Camera head captures the image based on the light received from the telescope. It converts light into information that is understood by electronic circuitry. Camera head consists of two parts viz. coupler and sensor. Coupler, as the name suggests, couples to the telescope. Sensor is responsible for converting light into image using sensors. These sensors are normally charged coupled devices (CCD) or more recently, complementary metal-oxide semiconductor (CMOS). CMOS scores better on light sensitivity, high speed, noise elimination and power consumption. Due to fabrication advantages of CCD, sometimes CCD scores better in uniformity and therefore better image quality. The differences between CCD and CMOS are summarised in Table 4.2.

The sensor can be a single chip sensor or a three chip sensor.

A single chip sensor, as sown in Fig. 4.6, reads all three colors where Green is the true color read by the silicon sensor and the Blue and Red are interpolated. In few other models, we find the blue and red and measured by physical line filters but not interpolated. Needs rephrase.

Table 4.2: Comparison between CCD and CMOS sensors		
Performance parameter	*CCD*	*CMOS*
Wavelength range	400–900 nm	350–1050 nm
Peak sensitivity at	Around 550 nm	Around 650 nm
Average sensitivity	Lower	Higher
Low light sensitivity	Higher	Lower
Saturation limits	Lower	Higher
Power consumption	Low	Much low
Dynamic range	Higher	Lower
Weight specifications	Heavier	Lighter

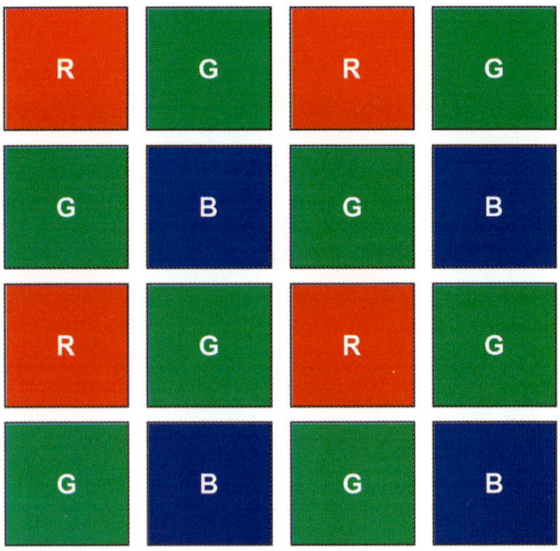

Fig. 4.6: Single chip camera uses mosaic filter and sense each primary colour by a different sensors in a pallet

In a 3 chip camera, the incoming light is split into three primary colours and then the sensors for each primary colour understand value of that colour component. The RGB values are then together used to understand the pixel value. There is one tiny sensor per pixel. The sensor plate consists of a matrix of these tiny sensors to capture the entire frame.

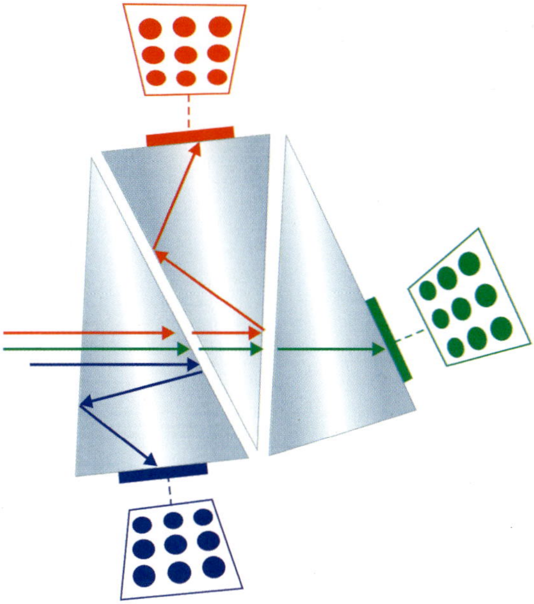

Fig. 4.7: Sensors in a 3-chip camera

Since the 3-chip camera, as shown in Fig. 4.7, captures the three primary colours individually, it gives image that is closer to the actual colours.

Camera head is characterised by frame size of the sensors, frame rate of the sensors, technology (CCD or CMOS), signal to noise ratio and light sensitivity.

Console Unit

Console unit receives images from the camera head in a suitable format. Console unit manages many controls. It processes the image for better clarity and uniformity. It also manages output to other devices including monitor and any recording device.

Video Cables

The connection between the console and the monitor decides the speed, frame size, frame rate and pixel depth.

Various types of cables and their characteristics are given in Table 4.3.

Table 4.3: Cable types and their characteristics

Cable type	*Brief description*	*Frame size*	*Frame rate*	*Pixel depth*	*Suitability for long distance*
DVI	Digital video interface/Transmitts uncompressed video-Modes- DVI-A analog and DVI-I digital and analog	2560 × 1600 for single line	30–85 Hz for single and 30–120 Hz for dual link	8, 12, 24 bits	No
HDMI	High definition multimedia Interface/proprietary audio, video interface to transmit compressed or uncompressed data.	2560 × 1600 single, 3840 × 2400 dual	25–120 Hz	8, 12, 24 bits	No
VGA	Videographics array/it can transmit uncompressed video modes–analog and digital and analog	2560 × 1600 single line	30–85 Hz	8, 12 bits	No
Composite with audio	Similar to DVI but capable of transmitting audio signal as well.	2560 × 600 single line 3840 × 2400 dual	30–85 Hz	8, 12, 24 bits	Yes
S video	Similar to HDMI	2560 × 1600 single, 3840 × 2400 dual	25–120 Hz	8, 12, 24 bits	No
Quad SDI	SDI category for HD and UHD.	HD, UHD	120 Hz	10–12 bits	Yes
12G SDI	SDI category for 2K, 4K and 8K	2K, 4K and 8K	30–60 Hz	10 bits	Yes

Monitor

Monitors display the live image. Monitors are characterised by the frame size, refresh rate, number of colours per pixel and the technology used. Also, monitors' physical dimensions are measured as the diagonal size in inches.

Typically the frame size is SD, HD or 4K.

Refresh rate is the ability of the monitor to refresh the current frame with the next frame as part of a video. Latest displays have refresh rates of 120 Hz, i.e. the display has the ability to display 120 consecutive frames within one second. The typical frame rate a.k.a. refresh rate is 60 Hz.

Typical pixel depth of monitors is 12 bit.

Most recent monitors can be based on technologies of LCD or LED.

While LCDs use diffusers and polarizers to obtain the contrast, LEDs use the ON OFF of diodes. Therefore, LEDs provide higher contrast, brighter, are more soothing to the eyes, are more colour rich and consume less power. LED displays have a longer lifetime as well.

Best Practices, Precautions and Troubleshooting

Use All Components from a Single Supplier

All the components of a camera system viz. telescope, console, CCD coupler, cables, light source and monitor from a single manufacturer are optimised for each other. So, using them from a single manufactuer gives best combined performance.

One can take liberty to use components from different manufacturers provided this aspect is understood and the choice of the components is conscious.

Quality of all the Components Needs to be of Roughly Same Level

Camera system is a series system and most of the components are in series. Each component in the system is capable of reducing overall quality but in most cases, does not have the ability to compensate for lack of quality of the other component.

Examples: If you have HD camera but the monitor is not HD, you will miss out on the quality of HD camera. If the light source does not provide enough light intensity, the monitor cannot compensate for it completely even though monitor has brightness setting. In many cases, a poor light cable can affect quality of image even though everything else is of great quality. Buying a 4 K image camera does not make sense unless the monitor is at least 32 inches.

So, when you are buying a full system, select components that provide roughly equal quality. Buying only one component of the highest quality typically does not improve the quality much.

Also, when you plan to upgrade your system in gradual manner, it is important to understand the bottleneck in the system and upgrade that item first.

Do Not Kink Fiber Cable

Fiber cable contains thousand of fibers. Fibers are delicate, each fiber being in microns in diameter. They can break if the fiber cable is kinked. Handling of the fiber cable should be careful to ensure that at no point in the cable, there is excessive pressure or kinking. While using or storing, maintain the circular shape, having diameter of no less than 8 inches, causing no acute angle at any point.

Avoiding Foggy Images

The distal lens of the telescope should be cleaned intermittently with irrigation, wiping with gauze before applying anti-fogging solution.

Ensure that the cannulas are clean and there is no tissue in the way while inserting the telescope.

Fogging of the telescope is a very common problem due to which the images look blurry and often miss out on most of the structures. To prevent the lenses from fogging, multiple methods were implemented. Most of the methods revolve around applying antifogging lotions or keep removing the telescope, clean it and navigate back to the location. While these methods work enough, these are not always feasible. Therefore, a few commercial devices use algorithm based software techniques such as filtering and denoising techniques to defog the images and a few other commercial systems use antifog plastics to cover the lenses.

Some insufflators have in-built warmer, which reduce fogging.

Care during Fumigation

Camera system components are delicate. Fumigation can cause deposition of the chemicals. Either keep these well covered or take them out of the OT during fumigation. This will enhance life of the product.

White Balancing

Red, green and blue (RGB) are the primary colours. Camera system is supposed to truthfully reproduce the same colours on the monitor as in the physical object. However, any one or more component(s) in the camera system can cause bias in weightage of these colours. For example, if the light source is more yellow than the noon sunlight, ultimately the image captured by the camera sensor will have more weightage to red and green because yellow is formed by combining red and green. The imbalance among the primary colours, caused by dominance of one or two primary colours, causes degradation in image quality.

White balance removes the imbalance in primary colours by counter-balancing them precisely. For the camera system to understand the imbalance, we need to provide a reference point to the camera system against which the camera system will check the balance. This reference is any white object, typically a gauze piece. Once the camera system gets the reference, it calculates the imbalance and applies counterbalance to the entire image. This correction is effective until the next time white balancing is done.

The best practices for white balance:

- At least 75–80%, if possible 100%, of the surface used for white balancing should be of white colour. Please do not used stained gauze piece.
- Whenever there is any change in the setup, white balancing should be done once again. This change in the setup could be

change of light source, cleaning of the telescope by betadine or dipping it in saline.

Placement of Monitor from Ergonomics Point of View

The monitor should be right in front of the surgeon. The distance between the surgeon and the monitor should be optimal. The desired distance is a function of monitor size, visual acuty of the surgeon. Also, the distance should not be so close to cause problem of convergence. Normally, the distance between the surgeon and the monitor should be 3–5 times of the diagonal length of the monitor, as shown in Fig. 4.8.

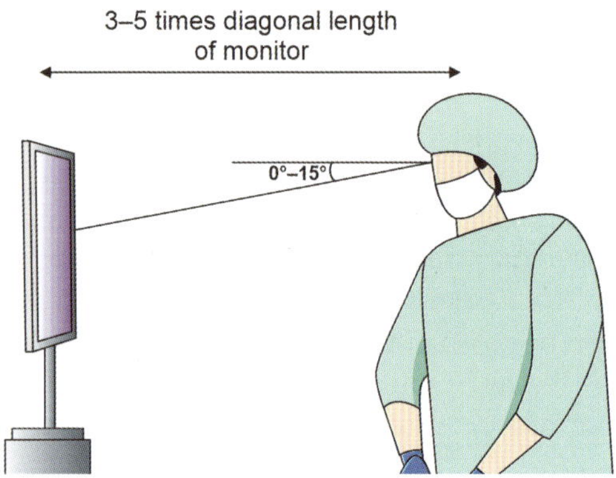

Fig. 4.8: Ideal ergonomics for monitor placement

As shown in Fig. 4.8, the monitor should be at 0–15 degrees downwards to avoid strain on neck of the surgeon.

Understand Programmability of Buttons on Camera Head

Modern camera heads have programmable buttons, which provide better control to the surgeon. The surgeon can program a specific button to a specific function e.g. recording of the video. It is advisable that the functions that are most frequently used or the functions that need to be used in a time critical manner, are programmed to the camera head buttons.

Optimal Setting

While the camera systems allow users to set the contrast, brightness, colour weightages for fine tuning the image settings, it is recommended to use the company provided settings based on the surgery. The settings for a laparoscopic surgery would be different from the settings for hysterescopic surgery. Most companies have preset settings for each of these types of surgeries and it is better to use the preset settings.

Sterilisation Methods

Follow sterilisation methods as recommended by the manufacturer, absence of which may lead to voiding of warranty and reducing life of the components.

Handling Video Cables

While inserting the video cables in the camera console port or monitor port, care should be taken to insert in the right port and ensuring inserting at the perpendicular angle. Else, the cables may get damaged or even the port may become loose.

Medical Grade Displays

Medical grade displays perform better than commercial displays in many ways. They are designed specifically for high-end requirements of surgery.

Brightness Remains Constant over a Longer Duration

Commercial displays lose brightness over time. Medical grade displays can measure the degradation and provide realtime compensation. Thus, the surgeons get consistent brightness over years.

A Wide Color Gamut

When the surgeon is not standing directly in front of the display, the colours seen by the surgeon should not change. In a medical grade display, colours do not change based on the viewing angle.

Faster Rendering

Fast rendering on the display is important for good hand-eye cordination. Medical grade displays have faster image processing so that the delay from the image capture to image rendering is minimal.

Noise Filters

Medical grade displays have noise filters that filter out electromagnetic noise which can cause distortion of images.

Easy to Clean and Disinfect

Surgical displays come without fan. The cooling happens through conviction and through vents. This reduces spread of contaminants.

Anti-glare Coating

The medical grade monitors come with anti-glare coating, which reduces reflection.

Professional Grade Connections

The medical grade monitors provide for professional grade connections like Quad SDI or 12G SDI as well. This allows for transfer of high quality images at longer distances.

Latest Trends in Optical Systems

3D Camera Systems

Two types:

- The active systems, where the images from each eye is processed independently to develop 3D images
- The passive systems where you require the polarization glasses to get the 3D effect. Each polarized images of various depths are mixed and then passively separated into the polarized glasses.

Wider the distance between the channels, more 3D effects

Humans can have depth perception and 3D vision because of two eyes, as can be seen in Fig. 4.9. The 3D systems allow great depth visualization and that allows surgeries to be performed with ease.

ICG

There are various dyes that can be injected in the body that stain certain types of cells. Surgeons are interested in understanding key landmarks, identify organ boundaries, locate vessels and

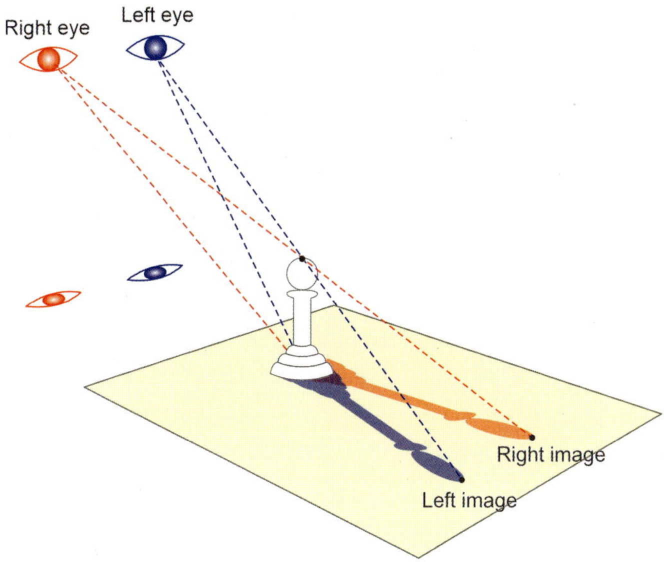

Fig. 4.9: Depth perception due to two eyes

blood flow. Indocyanine green (ICG) as a dye fits this requirement well because it binds with plasma proteins and thus targets lymph nodes and blood vessels.

Other advantages of ICG are:
- the low toxicity and nonionizing
- quick excretion, mostly into the bile
- flow limited to the vascular compartment
- depth imaging is possible because it works in tissue optical window
- ICG fluorescence is excited by infrared light, as shown in Fig. 4.10, which has a deeper penetration than visible light, allowing for visualization in deep tissue.
- As seen in Fig. 4.10, the fluorescence is generated by those structures that have blood flow, at around wavelength of 800 nm, where there is hardly any fluorescence from the tissue exists. This ensures quality of the fluorescence imaging.

The technology works as follows:
- ICG is injected intravenously and it gets into the vessels and other structures

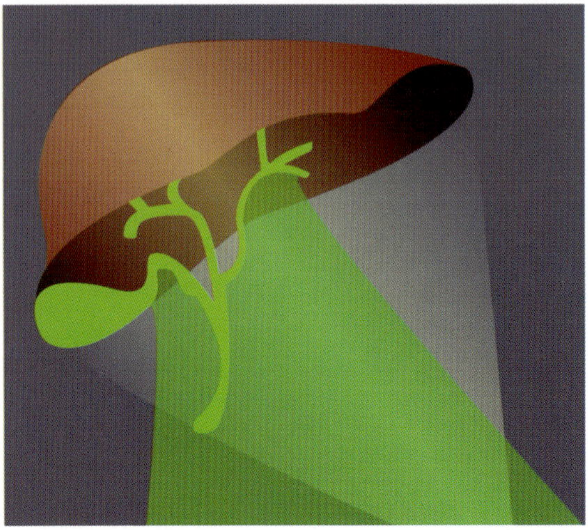

Fig. 4.10: Working of ICG

- Xenon light excites the ICG in blood flow and starts emiting fluorescence
- Camera has filter to separate the fluorescence light

The following changes are required in camera system compared to the regular camera:

- The light source should not have light in the fluorescence range otherwise, it will mix with the fluorescence emitted from the ICG dye.
- Camera sensor should be able to sense only the normal light or fluorescence by filtering out the other light.
- Alternatively, camera sensor should be able to sense normal light and the fluorescence individually and superimpose them on each other. This process is called as image registration and is a useful way so that we can relate the fluorescence intensity in the context of overall anatomy.

Uses of ICG

- Potentially preventing leaks as well as perfusion-related complications.
- Intraoperative real-time assessment of vascularization and tissue perfusion.

Disadvantages of ICG

- The cost of dye per surgery as well as the requirement of sophisticated camera system, particularly light source and camera sensor.
- ICG does not provide near real-time information about the blood flow.
- It requires approval of physician because ICG is contra-indicated in certain cases.

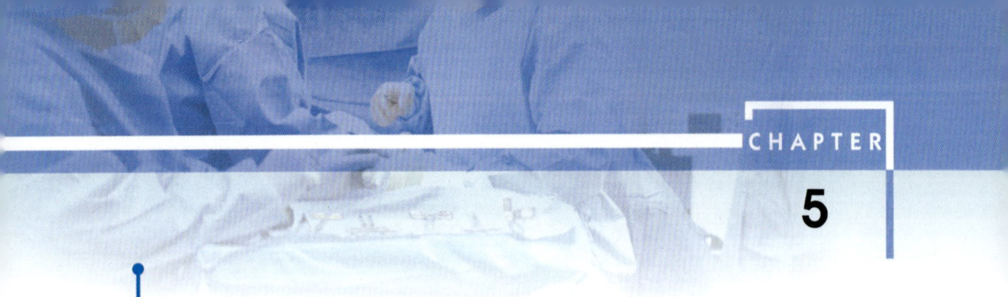

CHAPTER 5

Metal in Surgery

Girish Gangan

Metals used in surgery can be classified as per use, mainly:

1. Metals used in implants and
2. Metals used in instruments. Here we will be discussing in details about surgical instruments.

A surgical instrument is a tool or device for performing specific actions or carrying out desired effects during a surgery or operation. Surgical instruments plays a vital role in operation theatre along with the equipment. These are the tools used for any operation. Surgical instruments are categorised as per their usage. Nowadays, due to advancement in surgery the traditional instruments get modified or new instruments are invented. Minimally invasive surgery is encouraging the new dimensions of the instruments to be used and involves a lot of engineering skills to develop and manufacture the same.

Many countries have set stringent regulations, which need to be complied before someone markets or imports in that country. CDSCO, India has issued similar notification on September 3, 2020, mentioning classification of non-notified medical devices. Refer to www.cdscomdonline.gov.in for further details.

We will discuss following in this chapter:

1. Metallurgy used in surgical instruments
2. Types of surgical instruments
3. Selection criteria for surgical instruments
4. Use of surgical instruments in effective manner (covers do's and don'ts of material)

5. Storage and handling of instruments
6. Best practices for surgical instrument protection
7. Surgical instrument cleaning and Sterilisation methods

Metallurgy in Surgical Instruments

"Quality input is equal to quality output" is the basic principle that is applicable to all industries including medical devices. There are many considerations when it comes to selecting the right material to use in producing quality surgical instruments. Quality input for surgical instrument starts from basic raw material used, manufacturing processes involved and the verification of the final output before releasing to the customers. Selecting an incorrect input (material, manufacturing process and verification methods) may lead to serious consequences, e.g. infections, injury during surgery, post surgery complaints, etc.

Basic Properties of Material

Let us understand basic terminologies we come across related to metals.

- **Hardness** is ability of metal to resist plastic deformation induced by either indentation of abrasion.
- **Toughness** is ability of a material to absorb energy and plastically deform without fracturing.
- **Malleability** is the property of a metal to deform under compression and take a new shape without breaking.
- **Ductility** is metal's ability to drawing. In engineering term, it is defined by the degree to which a material can sustain plastic deformation under tensile stress before failure.

Among the above properties, it is important to distinguish between hardness and toughness. The differences are listed in Table 5.1.

Ductility vs Malleability

Ductility is the ability of a metal to undergo tensile stress, whereas malleability denotes the ability to undergo compressive stress.

So to begin with we will start with the materials used in surgical instruments manufacturing and the reasons of their usage.

When it comes to biomedical instruments, not all metals are up to the job, especially base metals. In fact, most surgical

Table 5.1: Difference between hardness v/s toughness

Hardness	*Toughness*
Hardenss is the resistance to cutting, abrasion and scratches	Toughness is resistance to fracturing. This depends on energy absorbed during fracturing.
Hardness depends on the strength and the plasticity of the material.	Toughness depends on ability of Material to be deformed under pressure. Tough material can withstand high pressure and are not easily breakable
e.g. Diamond is the hardest material Stainless steel is harder than titanium but titanium is tougher than stainless steel	e.g. Mild steel (popularly known as MS) is a tougher material, which is not easy to be cracked or broken

instruments are made from metal alloys. Stainless steel has traditionally been the metal alloy of choice, but there are alternatives when necessary.

First, the metal must be relatively flexible so it is often formed without causing defects, but not too soft because it must retain its shape once manufactured. Counting on the tool, the metal used must also be flexible, as many of the surgical instruments are long and thin, for example, consider the shape of curettes, scalpels, forceps, tongs, scissors.

The metal surface must be harsh and need a final touch of satin, so that the tools are easy to wash and do not contain bacteria. That way infections could be prevented from spreading. The metal must be inert with the physical body, so it may not cause any reaction due to the metal when it is used internally.

The most commonly used materials for surgical instruments are: Stainless steel, titanium, tantalum, platinum, palladium and tungsten carbide.

Various Metals Used in Surgery

Stainless Steel

Stainless steel or chromium steel is used for over 80% of the conventional surgical instruments produced worldwide in both types, the single-use, and re-usable instruments. Surgical steel

They are not hardenable via heat treatment but only by cold working (also known as work hardening). These steels have relatively low strength compared to the other steels and lower resistance to corrosion.

Austenitic stainless steels are split into two subcategories: the 300 series and 200 series. For the 300 series, the austenitic structure is achieved via the addition of nickel, whereas for the 200 series, this is achieved primarily via the addition of manganese and nitrogen.

Austenitic stainless steels are non-magnetic, however, the 300 series can become magnetic after cold working. The nickel content in the 300 series makes it suitable for low-temperature cryogenic applications.

Examples and applications of austenitic stainless steels:
304, the most common stainless steel contains 18 wt.% chromium and 8 wt.% nickel and therefore is often referred to as 18/8. 304 grade material is used for guide wires, graft punch, hammers etc where you need impact and not hardness in the instruments.

316, the second most common stainless steel, is used for example in implants. Instruments which does not require cutting or needs biocompatibility needs to made from this. Other example are food preparation equipment, chemical processing equipment, laboratory benches and equipment, heat exchangers and pharmaceutical and surgical equipment. Nowadays ISO 5832 compatible grade raw materials are available for implants as substitute to 316L (L represents low carbon content).

317, a low-carbon stainless steel with increased chromium, nickel and molybdenum for greater corrosion resistance. This is also used in implants for specific usage.

AISI 301 is the most commonly used metal for manufacturing springs which are useful in medical instruments. It gains mechanical strength when cold-worked, but loses corrosion resistance.

Martensitic: Martensitic stainless steels possess the body-centred tetragonal crystal system. They can range from having a low to high carbon content, up to 1.2 wt.%, contain 12–15 wt.% chromium and 0.2–1.0 wt.% molybdenum. They do not contain nickel. Due to the presence of carbon, they can be hardened via heat treatment, similar to carbon steels.

Martensitic stainless steels are magnetic and possess relatively high ductility and toughness, making them easier to form. They can be moderately hardened via cold working.

Higher carbon content results in increased strength and hardness but decreased ductility and toughness. They exhibit moderate corrosion resistance and poor weldability.

Examples and applications of martensitic stainless steels

410, used for highly stressed parts and used widely where corrosion is not severe–dental and surgical instruments, Bone holding clamps, holding instruments, retractors, etc.

420, is one of the most commonly used grade of stainless steel and has excellent wear and tear resistant due to higher carbon contains. Hence used for all cutting related instruments. In SS 420 there are various grades depending on composition of material by altering its alloy percentage, which gives different results (although it is termed as SS 420 grade only). Hence manufacturer's knowledge and its application makes huge difference in the material quality and careful selection of metal to manufacture surgical instrument. For 420, surgical drills, screw driver tips are the most common use. This grade is also used for cutlery, knife blades, surgical instruments, needle valves, shear blades, scissors and hand tools.

440, has very high carbon contains and higher hardness can be achieved after heat treatment, but is least corrosion resistance. hence used for cutting application where contact would be minimal. Storage of this grade in damped environment could cause rusting of the instrument and can cause rusting of other instruments as well.

Precipitation hardened steel is combination of austenitic and martensitic steels. It has higher toughness, strength and corrosion resistance. Grade 17-4 Ph stainless steel is most widely used steel of the precipitation hardening grade steels.

17-4 Ph is a special stainless used in surgical instruments, such as laparoscopic surgical devices. They are the grasping tools that are inserted through trocar. They can be grasper type (hold things) or cauterizing (burn and seal tissue).

Titanium

Titanium is right for both surgical instruments and implants because it is biocompatible and features a self-quality that blends well with human bones. For this reason, this metal has become the favourite for implants such as bone plates, bone screws, intramedullary nails, heart stents, dental implants, etc.

In general, titanium is a strong and sturdy metal that has become a standard material used for all types of medical purposes. The most obvious benefit of titanium is its superior strength. Its tensile strength is almost the same as carbon steel and it is 100% corrosion resistant. Despite its overall strength, it is more flexible than stainless steel and is approximately 40% lighter. Titanium is more resistant to heat than stainless steel, withstanding up to 430°C, and it expands and contracts less when heated and cooled.

The metal is immune to body fluids and is additionally highly resistant to corrosion, so it is often utilized in surgery without causing harmful effects. For equivalent reasons, they are also utilized in implants and bone replacement materials within the prosthesis.

Its usability is additionally a beautiful feature because it is often pulled into a skinny wire, while its malleability allows it to be easily manufactured in several forms.

Depending on the properties required for the instrument, titanium grade 1 or 2 can be machined, welded, and hot or cold-worked quite easily, so it is a versatile metal too. Addition of different alloys enhances different properties. Most common alloys additions are aluminium, vanadium and niobium for titanium.

In comparison with stainless steel, titanium is tougher material (can absorb more shocks), whereas stainless steel is harder material (can withstand more load). Titanium is more biocompatible than stainless steel, making its use versatile. But at the same time, application of instrument or implant would decide whether use of stainless steel vs titanium. In addition to the above properties, titanium is a more costly metal than stainless steel, hence cost factor has to be considered while deciding its usage.

Overall, titanium is a tough, durable metal that has become a common material used for all kinds of medical purposes.

Platinum and Palladium

Platinum and palladium are precious metals and expensive. Some unique properties make them the choice of metal in some limited number of surgical applications.

We can achieve any shape as well as precision that we need to form out of these metals, as they are flexible. Both platinum and palladium are corrosion resistant and inactive so that they are not reported as to cause problems when connecting to the body or internal organs.

Tungsten Carbide

Tungston carbide is very hard and brittle material. It is so brittle that if it falls on ground from hand it breaks into pieces. But due to its hardness it is used commonly in application areas such as tip of needle holders, cutting edge of scissors. These tips gives longer life of the instruments and wear and tear is much lesser.

Type of Surgical Instruments

The surgical instruments can be categorized by function:

- Cutting instruments include scissors, surgical blades, knives and scalpels.
- Retractors, which hold incisions open or hold an organ (or tissue) out of the way, include Gelpi, Weitlaner and US Army style instruments.
- Grasping or holding instruments include hemostatic forceps and tissue forceps.

In addition to the above-mentioned surgical instruments, we have many accessories available, which include all the extras needed for surgery. These include clamps, from large towel clamps to delicate vessel clips and bulldog clamps, drills, sutures, binocular loupes, biopsy punches and more.

Cutting Instruments

Scissors

Scissors are a piece of cutting instrument that has two sharp edges connected together at a centre so that the sharp edges glide against each other to shear material that is between the blades. Utilizing these sharp cutting edges, you can make fast, precise cuts with insignificant tissue harm. Examples of scissor are shown in Figs 5.1 and 5.2.

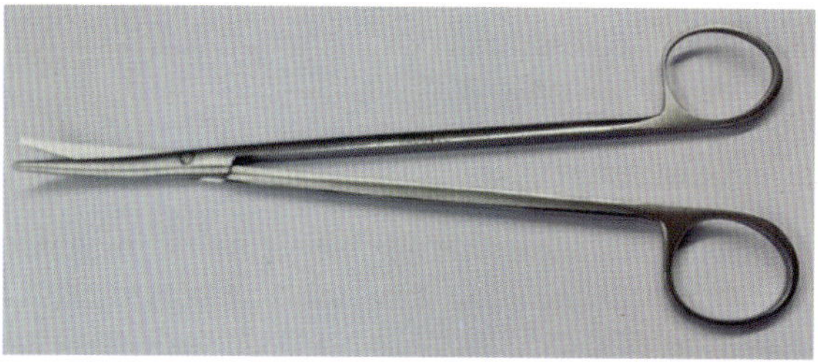

Fig. 5.1: S.S. scissor

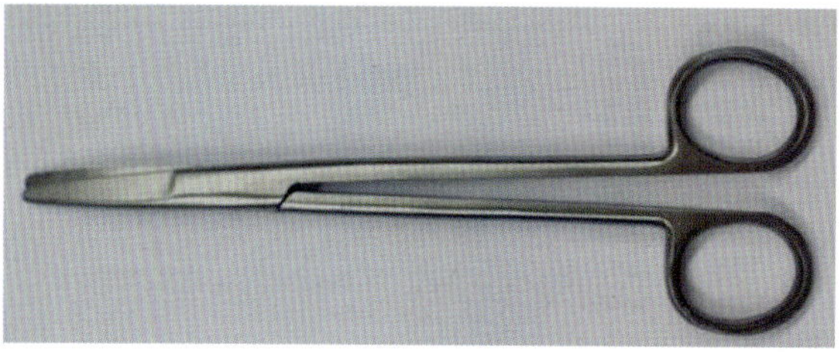

Fig. 5.2: Tungsten carbide tip scissor

Supercut scissors have one razor sharp blade and one micro-serrate blade. The sharp edge gives a clean cut with minimal tissue damage, and the serrated edge holds the tissue to prevent it from slipping while you are making an incision.

Here are some tips to keep in mind when selecting an appropriate pair of surgical scissors:

- Fine tip scissors (like Vannas, Castroviejos and McPhersons etc) are ideal for use in very restricted spaces. They are perfect for right or left hand use, and are designed for fine procedures, which require a delicate incision of tissue. You can make quick, accurate cuts with minimal tissue damage using these sharp blades.
- Curve tipped scissors are a good choice when you want to avoid cutting underlying tissues.
- Scissors designed with a heavier construction (like Metzenbaum, Mayo and SuperCut scissors) are useful for cutting fur, thicker tissue or vessels.

- The length of the scissor tips should match the depth of the incision. There are other cutting instruments. These include:
  1. Bone cutting instruments: Osteotomes, gouges, drills, saw blades etc.
  2. Wire cutting instruments
  3. There are various other cutting instruments as per their application.

Industry uses different types of steel for cutting applications. The cheapest option available is high carbon steel which has excellent cutting capacity but can not be considered as medical grade steel. High carbon steel usually gets rusted very easily due to its high carbon contents. All medical instruments when autoclaved, steam is passed at 120 degres over instruments. This causes rusting of the instruments and can spoil other instruments as well. Such rusted instruments can cause infections if it comes directly in contact with patients body. Therefore, high carbon steel wire cutters and pliers use should be avoided as much as possible.

Retractors

Retractors are the perfect option for opening an incision or open wound and holding the tissue to uncover what is underneath.

1. **Hand retractors:** An assistant, or the surgeon must hold hand retractors during a procedure, an example is shown in Fig. 5.3.
2. **Self-retaining retractors:** Self-retaining retractors have a mechanical gadget for holding tissue during a medical procedure, permitting without hands tasks. An example is shown in Fig. 5.4.

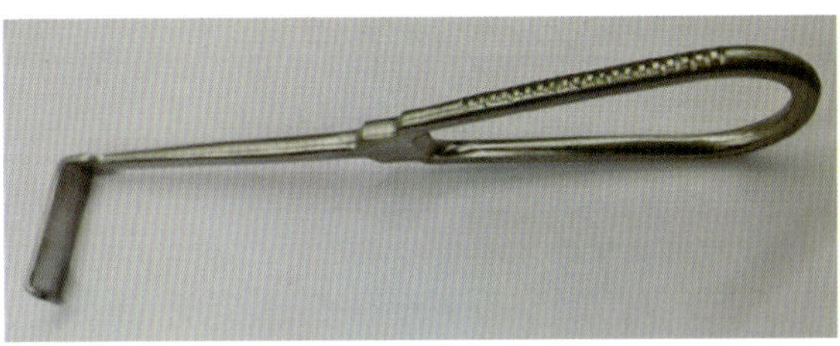

Fig. 5.3: Hand retractors

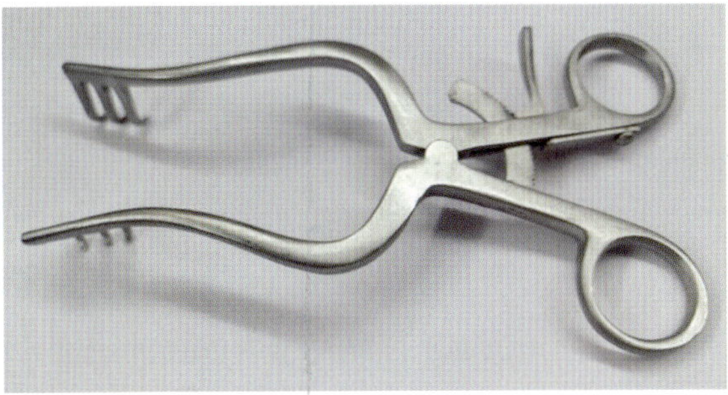

Fig. 5.4: Self-retaining retractor

3. **Wire retractors:** Wire retractors incorporate the wire that has some spring. The specialist can hold it together, position it and release it.

Grasping Instruments

The grasping instruments are designed for grasping tissue, tooth, bone, etc. as per type of surgery, e.g. disc forcep is used in spine surgery, meniscus grasping forcep in ACL surgery etc. Surgical forceps may be broadly divided into two categories viz. ring and thumb forceps (Figs 5.5 to 5.7).

The types of forceps are:

- Reverse forceps are self-closing. You squeeze them to open them. They provide uniform tension.

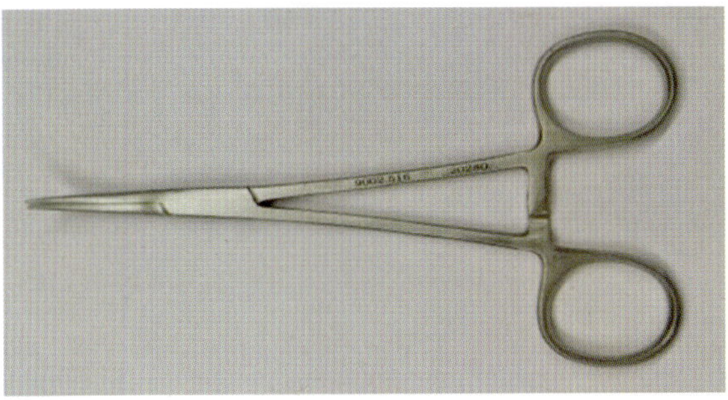

Fig. 5.5: Mosquito forceps

- Straight tips on forceps are used for general precision work, and slightly curved or fully curved tips provide more visibility.

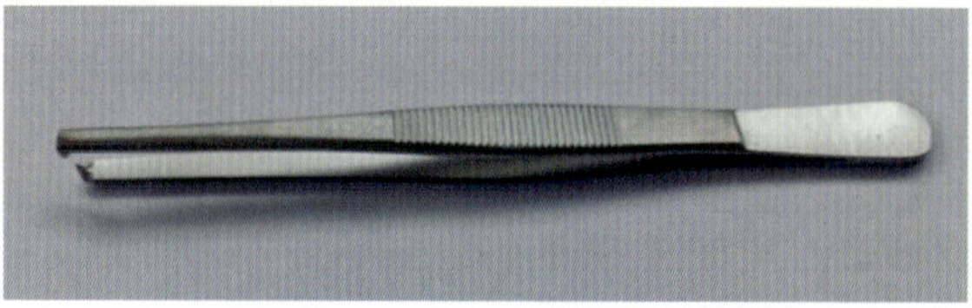

Fig. 5.6: Toothed forcep

- Ring forceps, also called locking forceps, are an instrument for grasping, holding firmly or exerting traction upon objects especially for delicate operations. They are hinged and look like ring scissors. Frequently, ring forceps have a locking mechanism called a ratchet, which is used for clamping. The jaws of the locking forceps gradually come together as each increment of the ratchet is employed.
- Thumb forceps are spring forceps used by compression between your thumb and forefinger and are used for grasping, holding or manipulating body tissue. They have no ratchet in the handle. Two broad categories of thumb forceps are dressing forceps and tissue forceps. Dressing forceps are used when dressing wounds and removing dressings. Very fine dressing forceps are also used in eye surgery. Tissue forceps generally have teeth, which offer a better grip on tissues while minimizing tissue damage.
- Toothed forcep (Fig. 5.6)

Selection Criteria for Surgical Instruments

How to Choose Appropriate Surgical Instruments?

Instruments would be reused over a long period of time. They also decide surgeons surgical skills and at times can prove to be lethal. Hence, spending quality time in selection of quality instrument is very important. It is also important to have reasonable expectations from the instruments.

When you are selecting surgical instruments for a procedure, here are a few key points to consider:

- What procedure are you performing? Published research papers usually indicate which instruments other researchers have used for similar procedures. The correct surgical

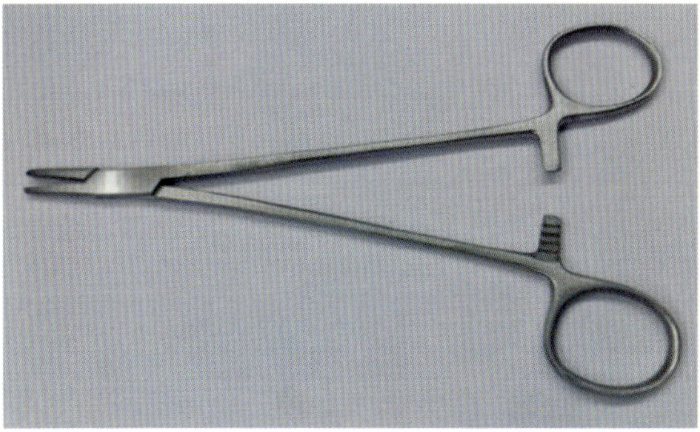

Fig. 5.7: Needle holder

instrument for a particular procedure makes a difference on the outcome of that technique.

- What is the size of your subject? An instrument that is perfect for an adult of 70–90 kg may not be the best choice for a neonatal or child of about 5–10 kg
- How often will the instrument be used? If you perform more than 100 cuts per day, a pair of titanium scissors or a pair of scissors with tungsten carbide inserts would be worth considering. They stay sharp longer.
- How ergonomic instruments are for your hand? Every surgeon has different hand. Ergonomically it makes a huge difference. Hence, selection has to be physical rather than just by referring to catalogs.

Other factors are:

Price: Quality instruments are different according to their price, which depends on the material from which the instruments are made.

Quality: Selectively invest in quality. Certain instruments, such as needle holders and scissors, are more likely to breed surgeon contention than others if quality or maintenance is sub par. Purchase the highest grade of these and similar instruments, and your surgeon and staff satisfaction will rise. Evaluate efforts by manufacturer for their quality acceptance criteria. It can be observed by careful inspection of instrument at the time of selection.

Material: Material selection is very important factor which depends on usage and application. This is mainly a part of manufacturers job. Hence, good technical knowhow of manufacturers management and staff is very important. Their qualification and experience makes a difference in selection of company or brand for purchase of instruments.

It is always important to remember the properties of material as discussed in previous section. Strong alloys such as titanium and stainless steel, as well as steel with chrome, nickel and molybdenum, provide a real guarantee against corrosion.

Sterilisation: Usually, the hospitals follow autoclave (steam sterilisation) as a preferred method for sterilisation. Instruments must necessarily withstand the necessary sterilisation treatment of various types, particularly autoclave. This factor is a direct proof of the high quality of the products.

Comfort: It is convenient for a doctor to work with instruments when they do not slip out of the hands, have a good grip, smooth contours that do not stick into the hand. The comfort component is the most important criterion when choosing instruments. This can only be achieved after in-person selection of instruments.

Streamlined purchasing: By focusing only on the instruments you need, you will save thousands of rupees. Sets are often designed by instrument companies and include unnecessary parts. For example, when buying a screw removal set, target only the necessary components and avoid sets having accessories which you never need. With reputed manufacturer, one tends to get technical knowledge as well as good instruments with after sales service which helps in streamlined purchasing.

Warranty of instruments: Always check for warranty of instruments and the reputation of supplier to keep their word for warranty of instruments. Remember that in order to fulfil warranty, the instrument should not be misused.

Use of Surgical Instruments in Effective Manner

Protection and careful handling of instruments saves money in the long run. It might increase your budget in the short run, but it will reduce your repair costs as well.

Surgical instruments are one of the largest assets of a hospital. Proper use of instrument protection devices and packaging aids can ensure costly surgical instruments are kept in top working condition.

The key to their longevity is proper care and maintenance. While stainless steel is universally regarded as the best material for surgical instruments, it is wrong to assume that it is absolutely corrosion-resistant. You need to remember that stainless steel instruments maintain their properties only with proper care. It is recommended that you always follow the manufacturer's instructions carefully and stick to these basic rules:

Use instruments for their intended purpose only: Incorrect or mixed use can damage the instruments beyond repair. For example, in practice, we have seen cutting instruments like nibblers used like pliers to pull wire, etc. Needle holders used as lever resulting in breakage of TC tip or bending of needle holder. Such things should be avoided.

Use of Instrument to its capacity mentioned by manufacturer: In cutting instruments its cutting capacity is mentioned many times on instrument or its description. If 2.5 mm wire is cut by using cutter of capacity of 2.0 mm, its life will decrease, or it would break.

Instruments should be cleaned and dried immediately after use. If they aren't, water and chemical residue will cause staining. Manufacturers recommend using distilled water and solutions with a pH below 10 for cleaning, rinsing, and Sterilisation. Always dry and Sterilise instruments in an open position. Take extra care not to damage fine tips and cutting parts.

Never use harsh solutions, abrasives, and steel brushes for cleaning and don't place instruments in saline: A nylon brush is effective for manual cleaning as long as you pay special attention to any hard-to-reach and moving parts.

Ultrasound cleaning is one of the most effective ways to clean surgical instruments. Do not forget to lubricate all moving parts after cleaning and before placing them in the autoclave. Be careful not to exceed the recommended exposure time when using disinfecting and Sterilising solutions.

In case of any breakage during use it is very important to convey correct information on how it happened to manufacturer, so that proper actions can be taken for improvement of instruments. Many times, false information leads to lapse of warranty and reduced confidence level between manufacturer and hospitals. Mal-handling or mal-usage of instrument should be conveyed.

Storage and Handling of Instruments

When it comes to instrument handling, care, and sterilisation, special emphasis must be placed on hospital staff education and training since fully functional and sterile instruments are critical to patient safety.

With highly specialized instruments and sets comes significant handling responsibility. Only necessary, highly qualified personnel should handle these types of instruments to ensure proper use and maintenance.

Label instruments wherever possible. Use indicator tapes. Nowadays, laser marking is another economical option for marking the instruments. The hospital or nursing homes initials can also be marked. Also to avoid mix up, set wise marking can be made in a short form.

Building smart trays from the start helps avoid the need to flash sterilise instruments. By keeping the selection and quantity to a minimum, you can use the base tray as a test to determine what needs to be added and what can be removed. Maintain instrument stock at a volume that anticipates days with high amounts of cases.

Rightsizing your existing trays allows for fast processing time, less work and lower cost. Carefully list all items in a tray and have a scrub tech track use for each item, creating new set lists when appropriate. Surgeons should review all updated trays and unused items should be removed. Only add to a tray when you are sure the instrument will be used in the majority of cases.

Remove rejected instruments from time to time. Depending on your department procedure, tag and remove rejected instruments from trays. Load instrumentation in a way to evenly disperse the weight in the tray. The total weight of the instrument set should not exceed 10–12 kg or a weight documented by the manufacturer of the Steriliser or container system.

Keep different sets of instruments and make a note of it. You can number the instruments by sets. The different sets can be marked differently.

Track by batch number of instruments. Usually standard manufacturing companies mark their batch number on instruments. Batch tracking helps in identifying the supply of instruments of the same batch to various customer to assess similar complaint.

The batch number traces instruments till its raw material stage and processes it involved to identify manufacturing defects. Batch numbers also help to track the life and usage of the instruments.

Create and maintain a detailed list of instruments in an electronic format preferably in ERP software or Excel. Include a complete instrument inventory, including specifics such as tray details and peel pack items. Nowadays many softwares provide support for inventory management and control.

Store your instruments in dry areas and make sure there are thoroughly dried before putting them into storage. Regular surface inspections and functionality checks are an essential part of the care routine.

Best Practices for Surgical Instrumentation Protection

1. Use containers to store instruments. If containers have specific space inside for each instrument laser marked them it makes sense to keep these instrument separately. It helps OT technicians for storage of instruments.
2. Wrap 'like-metals' such as copper/brass and stainless steel/chrome-plated instruments together, using tray liners or towels to separate them where necessary.
3. Wrap the smallest, delicate, and sharp-cutting instrumentation in woven or nonwoven towels, or other specially designed pouches. Use medical grade silicon ties to bundle instruments together and sterilise. Make sure the OR team knows which tip protectors are for which instruments. Rubber bands should not be used to hold instruments together. Usually in such mistakes company warranty may lapse and it would be a higher loss.
4. Store instruments with TC tip (Tungston carbide tip) separately. Tungston carbide is brittle by nature, hence if other

instruments fall on these or these instruments fall on the table or floor, they tend to break, making entire instrument useless. In such cases warranty lapses.

5. Store sharp instruments separately, as shown in Fig. 5.8. Use silicon tips to prevent cutting edges getting damaged.

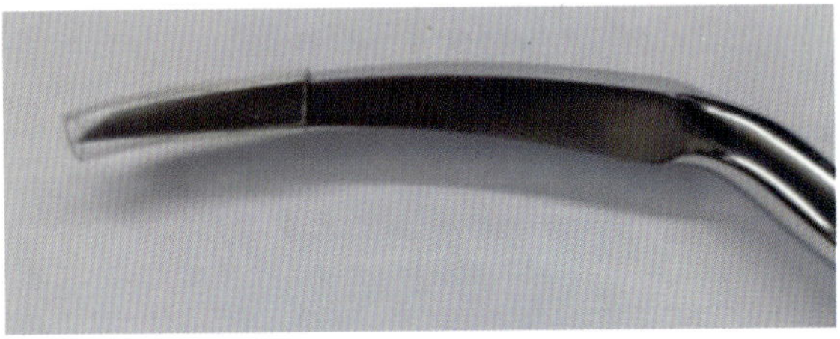

Fig. 5.8: Curved bone awl with protective silicon tip

6. *Observe stains on instruments:* Instruments usually if kept in contact with water tends to give rusting effect. Many times, it is superficial and can be cleaned by using alcohol or acetone with cotton or cotton cloth.

   Although stainless steel is corrosion resistant, it can still rust and/or stain if handled improperly. To determine if a discoloration is rust or just a stain, erase the discoloration with a pencil eraser. If there is pitting in the metal under the discoloration, it is corrosion. If the discoloration is removed, it was just a stain.

Stain color	*Cause*
Brown/orange	High pH of solution/water used for cleaning
Dark brown	Low pH of solution/water used for cleaning
Bluish/black	Reverse plating due to mixed metals during cleaning process
Multicolor	Material decolourisation due to excessive heat
Light/dark colored spots	Water droplets drying on the surface, not wiped after cleaning
Black	Contact with ammonia
Gray	Excessive use of rust remover solution
Rust	Dried on blood or biodebris and usually not in one place if material defect

7. High carbon steel instruments if in stock like industrial wire cutters after surgery should be cleaned and washed thoroughly to remove all blood stains and should be handled separately apart from other instruments. They need to be dried thoroughly. Best method of drying is by using air dryer. Air dryer keeps instruments in good conditions. Absence of water helps in longer life of instruments. The high carbon steel instruments need to oiled so that oxidation process can be prevented from moisture in air.
8. Keep instruments organized and open: Place ring-handled instruments on stringers, pins or racks to keep them open. Point clamps with curved jaws in the same direction to protect tips. Position cupped or concave instruments to avoid water collection.

   Use bunch clips wherever possible, as shown in Fig. 5.9. Bunch clips help in keeping the instruments organised and counting very easy especially of general instruments.

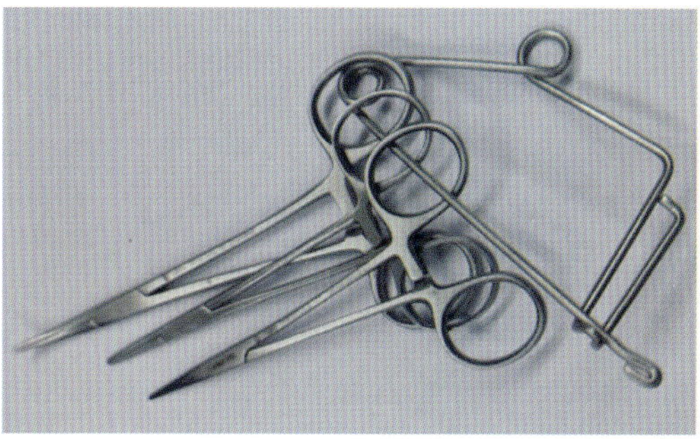

Fig. 5.9: Instruments in a bunch clip

9. Handle with care: Instrumentation should be carefully handled and removed from instrument trays and processing baskets. They should never be dumped onto work tables.
10. Involve your OR: The care of critical surgical instrumentation lies in the hands of the sterile processing technicians and the surgical team. Their attention to detail when following proper care and handling procedures will assure the safe use instrumentation, contributing to the best quality patient care outcomes.

Surgical Instrument Cleaning and Sterilisation Methods

The proper care and handling of your valuable surgical instruments will improve their longevity and function.

Choose a protocol appropriate for your environment from the cleaning method techniques below:

Rinsing

Immediately after use, rinse instruments under running water (preferably warm and not hot) to remove all blood, body fluids and tissue. Dried soils may damage the instrument surface and make cleaning very difficult. Do not use hot water as this will coagulate proteinous substances.

Cleaning Techniques

Time, temperature, and agitation play important roles in the cleaning process.

- **Time:** the efficiency of cleaning chemicals is often time dependent.
- **Temperature:** Higher temperature cleaning solutions result in better cleaning.
- **Agitation:** Whether manual or ultrasonic, it is helpful in loosening the soil on the surface of the instrument

Ultrasonic Cleaning

Ultrasonic is the most effective cleaning method. Ultrasonic cleaning is the result of cavitation. Vibrating sound waves create micron-size bubbles in solution that grow with the alternating pressure. When they reach a resonant size, the bubbles implode creating a force that dislodges dirt and particles, even in the smallest of crevices. Use of ultrasonic detergent greatly improves the cavitation rate as opposed to plain water.

Procedure of Ultrasonic Cleaning

1. Mix enzymatic (Enzol), or other neutral pH or mild alkaline detergent (Alconox) per manufacturer recommendations.
2. Use deionized water, if available.
3. Run ultrasonic cleaner for several minutes to degas the solution and obtain correct temperature.

4. Place instruments in open position into the ultrasonic cleaner. Do not allow instruments with sharp blades to touch other instruments. All instruments must be fully submerged.
5. Do not place dissimilar metals (stainless, copper, chrome plated, etc.) in the same cleaning cycle.
6. Instruments should be processed in cleaner for 5–10 minutes.
7. Rinse instruments with water to remove ultrasonic cleaning solution and any remaining soils.
8. Dry instruments thoroughly with a clean towel or air spray. This minimizes the risk of corrosion and formation of water spots.
9. Use spray lubricant in the hinges to improve function of instrument.

Manual Cleaning

1. Use stiff plastic cleaning brushes. Do not use steel wool or wire brushes.
2. Use only neutral pH detergents. If not rinsed properly, low pH detergents may breakdown the stainless protective surface and cause black staining. High pH detergents may cause surface deposits of brown stains, which can interfere with the smooth operation of the instrument.
3. Brush delicate instruments carefully and, if possible, handle them separately from general instruments.
4. Inspect all instrument surfaces to ensure they are visibly clean and free of stains and tissue. Inspect each instrument for proper function and condition. Scissor blades should glide smoothly and the blades must not be loose when in closed position. Check that forceps tips are properly aligned. Hemostats and needle holders should not show light between the jaws, they should lock and unlock easily, and the joints should not be too loose. Check needle holder jaws for wear. Examine cutting instruments and knives to be sure their blades are sharp and undamaged.
5. Rinse instruments thoroughly under running water. While rinsing, open and close scissors, hemostats, needle holders and other hinged instruments to ensure that hinge areas are also rinsed.
6. Dry instruments thoroughly with a clean towel. This minimizes the risk of corrosion and formation of water spots.

Soaking

Large, non-delicate instruments can be soaked in a corrosion inhibiting detergent (Alconox etc.) when other cleaning methods are not practical. Rinsing and drying after soaking is recommended.

Sterilising Methods

Choosing a sterilisation method is one of the most important steps in medical device. At worst, poor sterilisation can lead to transmission of infectious diseases causing patient illness and even death.

A number of both physical and chemical processes can be used to properly sterilise a medical device, however steam sterilisation, dry heat sterilisation, chemical sterilisation using gases like ethylene oxide, and radiation are among the most common.

Physical or Chemical Medical Device Sterilisation

A number of both physical and chemical **processes** can be used to properly sterilise a medical device; however, steam sterilisation, dry heat sterilisation, chemical sterilisation using gases like ethylene oxide, and radiation are among the most common. The choice of sterilisation technique will depend on the material composition of the medical device, how it is classified, and its intended use.

It is important to distinguish between sterilisation and cleaning. Without first cleaning away any debris from surfaces, and in the case of gaseous sterilisation thoroughly drying the surfaces, medical devices cannot be properly sterilised. In the case of disposable medical supplies such as syringes and scalpels, impurities deposited during the manufacturing process must be removed before the devices are packaged and sterilised.

This pre-sterilisation cleaning process becomes even more important when it comes to reusable devices like endoscopes and other surgical instruments such as clamps and forceps. The accumulation of blood, tissue and other contaminants significantly limits the ability of sterilisation procedures to properly eliminate microorganisms, and most importantly pathogens, from these reprocessed devices and tools.

Packaging, transportation and storage conditions should also be considered when choosing a method of medical device sterilisation. Products designed to be aterilised directly prior to being used on a patient will require less-stringent handling protocols in the supply chain. In contrast, those devices designed to arrive at the healthcare facility pre-sterilised should be packaged in such a way as to maintain that sterility while minimizing the device's exposure to fluctuations in temperature, humidity and airborne particulates. Instruments should be stored in a clean and dry environment until use after sterilising.

Steam Sterilisation

Steam sterilisation is most appropriate for devices composed of stable, heat-resistant materials such as steel, characterized by high temperatures and pressures. Reusable surgical tools are often steam sterilised in an autoclave to kill any microorganisms that may be present on the surface of the instruments, as well as bacterial spores, which can be resistant to other forms of disinfection. It is a quicker and less costlier method to have in house sterilisation. While the steam sterilisation process itself takes just 15–60 minutes cycle at 121°C depending on type and manufacturers recommendation, medical instruments must be allowed to cool and dry completely over the course of several hours before being used.

Steam sterilisation is sometimes not the decontamination method of choice for medical device manufacturers due to:

1. The build up of water droplets inside device components can impair their functioning and corrode materials that are not meant to come into contact with water.
2. Plastic and electronic components can also be damaged by exposure to steam or higher temperature, making this sterilisation method unsuitable for most complex medical devices.

Instructions to be followed for autoclave sterilisation:

1. Instruments may be autoclaved individually or in sets. Place heavy instruments on bottom of set (when two layers are required).

2. Never lock an instrument during autoclaving. This will prevent the steam from reaching and sterilising the metal-to-metal surfaces. Furthermore, heat expansion during autoclaving can cause cracks in hinge areas.
3. Do not overload the autoclave chamber, as this may also hinder steam penetration.
4. Place a towel on bottom of pan to absorb excess moisture during autoclaving.
5. At the end of the autoclave cycle (before the drying cycle) unlock autoclave door and open it no more than a crack (about ¾″). Run dry cycle for the period recommended by the autoclave manufacturer. If the autoclave door is opened fully before the drying cycle, cold room air will rush into the chamber, causing condensation on the instruments. This will result in water stains on instruments and also cause wet packs.

Cold Sterilisation

If the instruments need only to be disinfected (basically clean), cold sterilisation is acceptable since disinfection will take place in only 10 minutes. But to render the instruments sterile (with absolutely no living organism surviving), autoclaving is recommended. Most cold sterilisation solutions require a 10-hour immersion to render instruments sterile, but this prolonged chemical action may be more detrimental to surgical instruments than the 20-minute autoclave cycle. For instruments with tungsten carbide inserts (needle holders, scissors, tissue forceps), do not use solutions containing benzyl ammonium chloride which will destroy the tungsten carbide inserts.

Dry Heat Sterilisation

Dry heart sterilisation takes longer than steam sterilisation due to the inefficiencies of heating air with a very low moisture content. Compared to steam sterilisation, which requires a temperature around 121°C to be maintained for approximately 30 minutes, dry heat Sterilisation requires higher temperatures of around 180°C to be effective at neutralizing biological contaminants and their spores. For this reason, dry heat sterilisation is most appropriate for medical devices which are heat resistant but susceptible to water damage which would make steam sterilisation a poor choice. Hot air ovens are the most common setup for dry heat sterilisation of tools composed of metal or glass. Vials containing biologic drugs such as vaccines are often sterilised using a dry heat method prior to filling to ensure they contain no microorganisms.

Ethylene Oxide Sterilisation

Ethylene oxide sterilisation is a chemical method that is popular among medical device manufacturers. Unlike steam sterilisation and dry heat sterilisation which require that the medical device be heat stable, a variety of materials—like plastics and electronic components—can be exposed to ethylene oxide gas without distorting the medical device's form or ability to function.

As an alkaline agent, ethylene oxide gas reacts with DNA, proteins and enzymes to disrupt cell growth and division, thereby killing the microorganism. In addition to being able to penetrate small spaces inside medical devices, ethylene oxide can also be used to sterilise medical devices that have already been packaged in plastic.

However, this method of medical device sterilisation does have its drawbacks; for one, ethylene oxide gas is toxic to humans and highly reactive at low temperatures, making it imperative that the sterilisation procedure take place in a leak-proof chamber. In addition, the method is more complex compared to other forms of sterilisation as it requires three steps to complete. First, devices are prepared for sterilisation through environmental controls, then, the operator sterilises the device through the addition of the gas, and finally, the gas is thoroughly removed from the product.

Radiation Sterilisation

Sterilisation of medical devices using radiation does not leave behind any trace radioactivity, therefore, irradiating medical devices using gamma or electron beam (E-beam) radiation is a clean way to sterilise.

Like ethylene oxide sterilisation, radiation can penetrate product packaging. However, the latter is a less time-consuming method. Dense materials can also be irradiated quite efficiently.

This sterilisation technique is best-suited to single-use devices like implants, catheters and syringes. When used to sterilise reusable devices, processors will need to perform quarterly dose audits to ensure that the level of radiation exposure is sufficient to destroy any microorganisms on the device.

This Sterilisation method causes little fluctuation in temperature, making it appropriate for use on devices made from heat-sensitive plastics and other materials. Pre-filled syringes and other disposable medical devices can be Sterilised using this method. However, care must be taken when using this method as it can cause cosmetic and functional issues such as discoloration, and deleterious effects on various materials used in the device.

Verifying Medical Device Sterilisation

Once you have chosen one of the above sterilisation techniques that best suits your medical device, you will need to validate that the method is properly sterilising the device. One of the ways to accomplish this is by testing device surfaces for the presence of any microorganisms. The choice of an appropriate sterilisation technique can make a difference in the lives of patients.

CHAPTER 6

Upcoming Technologies

Sudarshan Nagaonkar

Practioners and innovators have always strived to make the surgery safe, bring consistency and improvement in clinical outcomes. The innovations include surgical technique as well as involvement of better technology. While there are many streams of developments that are taking place, in this chapter, we will cover a few technologies with brightest prospects, viz. robotics, artificial intelligence, AR and VR and 3D printing.

For each of these technologies, we will cover fundamentals, broad application areas, advantages of the technology and current limitations.

Robotic Surgery

As per Wikipedia:

Robotics is an interdisciplinary research area at the interface of computer science and engineering. The goal of robotics is to design intelligent machines that can help and assist humans in their day-to-day lives and keep everyone safe.

Robotics develops machines that can substitute for humans and replicate human actions.

Robotic surgery has been in existent for more than 20 years. The first trans-altanic robotic surgery was successfully done in 2001.

Robotic surgery is not a surgery done by robot but it is a surgery done by the surgeon with the help of robotic arms. It is highly advanced technology covering medical optics and robotic instrumentation.

Currently, there are broadly two specialties where robotic surgery is being used, viz. laparoscopy and orthopaedic.

The robotic surgery system for laparoscopy is used for all the activities right after port insertion till just before ports are removed.

The system for orthopaedic surgeries like knee replacement, the system takes CT scan data and helps the surgeon in planning the surgery. Also, the system is part of the surgery setup for ensuring that precisely those parts (bones, tissues) are removed as planned and helps in precise placement of implants.

Robotic Surgery for Laparoscopy

Typically, the robotic surgery system consists of the following:

- Surgeon console
- Patient side cart
- Instrument set
- Vision cart

Surgeon Console

Surgeon console is the place where the surgeon sits and operates the robotic system. The console consists of 3D high definition display, master controls that are operated by hands and footswitches that are operated by foot.

The display also provides information like type of instruments being used, type of energy source connected, orientation of the camera.

Master controls allows finger movements into real-time movement of the instruments. Typically, only three fingers viz. thumb, index finger and middle finger are used for control of the instruments.

The foot pedals are used for controling camera (positioning, orientation and focus) and activation of energy source.

Patient Side Cart

Patient side cart supports robotic arms, typically three or four. The robotic arms carry out surgeon's commands. The cart is docked by bringing it over the patient to a center post. The docking happens with reference to trocars. The arms are referenced to a fixed pivot point i.e. trocars as result of docking. One arm is used for camera while other arms are used for instruments.

Instrument Set

The instrument is designed to replicate the surgeon's hand and wrist movements. In fact, the ability of the instrument goes beyond the human wrist and the instrument set has seven degrees of freedom. This gives better maneuverability compared to wrist movement and traditional instruments. The instrument set will consists of variety of instruments based on purpose e.g. dissecting, suturing, grasping, cutting, coagulating, stapling, sealing and ultrasonic energy instruments.

Vision Cart

Vision cart has high definition 3D camera that sends images continuously to the surgeon console. It also has a 2D display that shows the same images seen by the surgeon, except that it is 2D. It also shows the same set of information that is visible to the surgeon, i.e. instruments being used, type of energy source connected, orientation of the camera. The 2D display is utilised by the clinicans on the patient side.

Advantages of the Robotic Surgery

- **Precision:** Precision in robotic surgery is result of many technologies. The high definition 3D image allows the surgeon to target the tissue better. The instructions from the surgeon console gets transferred to the instrument set. During this transmission, the advanced algorithms remove the tremors and smoothen the movement. The fine control of movement is possible by changing the movement amplification factor. The seven degrees of movement allow for precise placement in the right direction.
- **Surgeon ergonomics:** A high percentage of surgeons regularly feel musculoskeletal pain related to work and that they have twice the risk of such injuries as the general population. In one of the recent studies, surgeons rated their pain at close to 5 out of 10 at the beginning of a surgery day and 7 or 8 by the end. Seating operating posture, monitor at the level of eyesight, resting for wrists and easy controls reduce surgeon fatigue drastically.

- **Better patient outcomes:** Patients get faster recovery, shortened hospital stays, less post operative pain and reduced complications. These are result of precision and high definition 3D images the surgeon gets.
- **Remote surgery is possible:** Even though the most commonly the surgeon console is in the same room or premise where the patient is, it is possible for a surgeon to perform surgery remotely. In fact, the first transatlantic surgery was done in 2001. With the advent of 5G, the latency and speed of communication will be far better than 4G wireless technology. This will allow, for example, surgeons in the city to perform surgeries on patients in rural set up without having to travel. Many robotic systems have facility of double console. At any point of time, one console is in control while the other control is in observation mode. The control can be switched between the consoles at any time. The main use case of the double consoles is to train surgeons. In the future, it will be possible for an expert surgeon to be available remotely through his/her console, which can be in observing or controlling mode.
- **Learning curve:** Every new technology with it brings its own set of context and mechanisms. A certain amount of learning, unlearning and relearning is required to adapt to robotic surgery. Till that is achieved, the optimal results are not possible.

  Having said that, it has been observed that learning curve for robotic surgery is faster compared to laparoscopic surgery.

Limitations of the Robotic Surgery

- **Lack of tactile feedback:** Surgeons are used to tactile feedback, which does not exist in robotic surgery. The surgeon needs to rely only the visual mechanism to get feedback from the surgery field.
- **Cost:** The one time cost is very high. Also, most of the instruments are disposable instruments increasing recurring cost also drastically.

Robotic Surgery for Orthopaedic

The system for surgeries like total knee replacement entails the planning and execution phases.

3D Planning Phase

Input to the system is CT scans. The system creates a 3D model of the bones. The surgeon decides how much bone to be cut and where. The surgeon explores various implant sizes, orientation and placement. Once all the decisions are confirmed, the planning phase is complete.

Robot-assisted Execution Phase

During the surgery, the first step for the robot is to understand the landmarks. These are done with the help of landmark calibration. This helps the robot to correlate the CT scan data with the actual patient data.

Based on load balancing parameters, the robot calculates how much bone should be cut and where. These are graphically displayed on the display.

The guidance is available to the surgeon continuously while the surgeon cuts the bone by the tool attached to the robotic arm. This ensures that the bones are cut only as much as needed. If the surgeon cuts extra bone even by 1 mm, that is indicated as well.

During placement of the implant, the software indicates if there are any deviation compared to the planned placement. This helps the surgeon in precise placement of the implant.

Minor adjustments are always within the control of surgeon.

Benefits of the Robotic Surgery for Orthopaedic

1. Precise placement of implant is possible
2. Bone is cut only as much as needed and not more
3. Postoperative pain is less compared to the manual methods
4. Recovery is faster for the patient
5. Less possibility of revision surgery due to higher precision
6. Reduced blood loss during surgery

Augmented Reality

Augmented reality is when computer-generated image is superimposed on the physical world. Thus, the physical world is complemented by the information that is computer generated. Also, the information generated is contextualised with respect to the physical world. The information is played in realtime.

Since the information is overlayed on the physical world, there is no need to takes the eyes off the surgical site.

Computer processes data received from various sources and generate the image. This process is specific to each augmented reality application.

Applications of Augmented Reality

Given below are just some of the applications of augmented reality to give you an idea of what is possible:

- **Organ, landmark and blood flow identification:** A computer identifies organs, landmarks and blood flow during a surgery. This information is displayed by colour coded annotation on top of the image shown on the display by the laparoscopic camera.
- **Tumour boundary identification:** An onco surgeon is wearing a smart glass during an open surgery for tumour removal. During the surgery, the tumour is highlighted by the smart glass, clearly indicating tumour boundaries. The smart glass has this information from the CT scan with reference to some neutral landmarks and is thus able to identify tumour boundaries precisely.
- **Remote proctoring:** An expert surgeon can log in from remote and has access to the live video. He also has a console where he can point to the specific landmarks and can speak on the microphone.

The proctoree sees the expert surgeon's 'hand' on the secondary screen, which points the landmarks or the plane. The proctoree is also able to hear what the expert surgeon says. This 'hand' is an example of augmented reality.

Virtual Reality

In our normal course of life, we are conscious of our physical environment. For example, we are watching a cricket match on TV at home. While our mind is focused on the match, we are still conscious of our home environment at back of our mind. However, if we are inside a stadium, the experience is fullsome. For example, if we want to observe a specific player, we can do that. Our senses absorb more in such an environment.

Such memories are long lasting and also our acquisition of understanding is deeper. Also, you are not just an observor but also a participating in fullsome experience.

Virtual reality tries to provide this fullsome experience with these additional benefits.

- Virtual reality provides computer generated immersive environment for the user to feel it close to reality. In virtual reality, the environment itself is the experience and the user is virtually transported inside the environment.
- Extending the above analogy, in our physical reality, if we wish to enjoy a specific cricket match, it has limitations in terms of space and time. It means the stadium size has a limit and we need to attend that match on that specific day.

Virtual reality overcomes these limitations.

- Virtual reality systems typically consist of headgears that provide visual information to the user in 3D. They may additionally contain hardware gears that are specific to a particular application. For example, flight simulators have panel that resembles the control panel of an aircraft.
- Virtual reality has immense potential in training of surgeons. It is scalable, i.e. it can train a large number of surgeons, simultaneously or at different times. It is possible for the surgeons to perform complete surgeries or the key steps like suturing in the virtual world. These can be repeated until the learning curve is achieved. Since it is the virtual world, they are safe and do not have much recurring costs. Since the actions of the trainee are captured by the system, it is possible for the system to provide a rating immediately without using time of the proctor.

Artificial Intelligence

There are many tasks than computers can do well with speed and accuracy. For example, multiplication of two large numbers. Conversely, there are many tasks that human beings are good at. For example, holding a conversation, reading hand written text.

Artificial intelligence (AI) is a branch of computer science dedicated to machines that are designed to perform activities that human beings are typically good at, without being explicitly programmed. The current AI systems are specific to narrow scope of work. For example, automated driving, speech recognition.

There are many techniques by which AI system is achieved including deep learning, expert systems. Deep learning is the most common technique used in AI.

Deep Learning

Deep learning technique is based on neural networks and thus broadly mimics how human brain works. The difference is that human brain has tens of billions of neurons. For deep learning, such high number of neurons is neither practical (due to limitations of computation power) nor required for learning a specific task (while human brain learns any number of tasks).

Deep learning works by:
- Input to output mapping is given the AI system
- Based on a large set of input-output values, the AI system learns the relationship
- When a new input comes, the system infers output.

For example, deep learning engine can be trained by images (input) of various birds and their names (output). Once trained, if you any input picture of a bird, it will infer name of the bird.

The inference actually is in the form of percentage of confidence on each of the options. For example, the system may say that an image is of Crow at 92% confidence and of Common Raven at 8% confidence.

Applications of AI in Surgery

Given below are just some of the examples that demonstrate the possibility of using AI in surgery. The applications depend on the suitability and also creative thinking.
- **Identification of smoke during laparoscopic surgery:** AI system can be used to identify presence of smoke during surgery. Once the system recognises presence of smoke, the insuflator gets changed for high flow automatically. Once the smoke is gone, the insuflator reverts to regular flow rate.
- **Understanding phases of a surgery:** AI systems have been used to identify phases of a surgery and thus the AI system can calculate time taken by a surgeon for each phase

of surgery. This can help a surgeon to understand his/her progress for each phase of the surgery.

- **Prediction of risks:** AI systems have shown remarkable results in predicting risks and outcomes. For example, prediction of pancreatitis severity 6 hours after admission or anastomotic leaks of postoperative colorectal patients. It is possible to come out with a surgery specific post surgery risk analysis by taking various factors (patient history, vital signs, medical records, key images during surgery) into account.
- **Feedback on surgery:** AI system can provide specific feedback on each step of the surgery, just by analysing the surgery video. The feedback can also mention how a KOL recommends performance of the step.
- **AI based robotic surgery:** Small tasks like suturing can be performed autonomously using robotic arms. The futuristic scenario is where entire surgery is completed autonomously using robotic platform though it will take decades for such a system to come into existence.

Advantages of AI

- **Expertise of the top professionals available to wider user base:** AI systems work on the foundation of data. The data is collected from the best experts in the domain. Thus, this expertise is available to wider users. In effect, expertise of the top professionals get captured in usable form and is made available.
- **No fatigue:** AI systems, being machine based, do not have fatigue, cannot get tired and are available for 24 hours a day. Also, they provide consistent output without being affected by factors that affect human professionals.

Limitations of AI

- **Explainability of inference:** In most cases, AI will provide inference but will not be able to explain the inference. This can be problematic in medical domain. Even though studies have shown better accuracy by AI compared to professionals, lack of explainability makes it less credible. For example, if a professional makes a certain diagnosis, it is possible to ask for explanation and have a discussion. And the professional can change the diagnosis after a meaningful discussion. Such option is not available with AI. So, even if AI has better accuracy, in the event the inference is in doubt, there is no recourse available.

- **Results depend on good data:** AI needs large number of data, while humans can learn based on just a few examples. If the data has errors, any bias; then the inferences will carry those biases and errors in it.

  Also, if any new scenario is arisen, AI systems are not good at providing inferences. This can be considered as lack of good data but sometimes, new unique situations do arise.

Autonomous Surgery

When technologies like advanced vision, AI and robotics come together, they can make autonomous surgery possible. The first autonomous robotic soft tissue surgery (porcine intestinal anastomosis) was conducted in 2016. It demonstrated superior performance compared to human surgeon for suturing task. The task is typically considered difficult for robots given tissue deformity and mobility.

3D Printing

3D printing is a new way of manufacturing. It is a type of additive manufacturing. The regular manufacturing typically involves series of steps and in each of the steps, some material is removed by way of machining processes until the desired specifications are achieved.

In 3D printing, a layer is added at a time. When all the layers are added, the desired specification is achieved.

First the user needs to convert the 3D model into slicing information. This is done by 3D design file and other inputs like layer height, speed. The output of this process is a gcode file, which contains slicing information.

The 3D printer takes the G-code file, calculates where the material should be used at each of the layer and prints it layer by layer. For example, if height of the part is 50 mm and each layer it 0.1 mm, there will be 500 layers.

A 3D printer consists of heater that melts material used for printing, extruder nozzle that lays the material and computer programmed robotic motion that decides movement of the nozzle and switches on and off the material flow based on the design. Once a layer is complete, the nozzle is lifted by height of one layer. By the time the nozzle comes back to the same position, albeit at a one layer height above, the material solidifies already.

There are less common methods which include laser based technology for melting metals and those work upside down, i.e. top layer is formed first.

When the 3D printing was new, the accuracy was not good. So, they were mostly used for prototype. Now, the lowest layer height possible is 0.05 mm. However, lower height leads to longer time to print.

Also, there was limitation on the type of material used. Earlier, only polymers were being used but now, 3D printing of metal is possible as well. Polylactic acid (PLA) is the most commonly used polymer. Recently, silicon is also being used for 3D printing though it is not very common.

Advantages of 3D Printing

- **No non-recurring expenses:** Most of the manufacturing, particularly those that require objects that are not simple, require development of tools. The tools cost can be range from a few thousands of rupees to a few lakhs of rupees, depending on the complexity of the part and cost optimisation required at per unit cost. This can be prohibitively high for some applications.
- **Complex shapes, hollow parts possible:** Traditional manufacturing methods are not easily ameneable to complex shapes or hollow parts. For 3D printing, this is not a challenge and it is equally easy for it as a routine shape is.
- **Manufacturing can be at the last mile:** Many product companies are exploring an option to share 3D printable model of their spare parts with their dealers. In such a scenario, the dealer does not need to keep stock and can simply print the spare part on demand using a 3D printer.

Applications

Specimen Models for Surgeries like Orthognathic

When the surgeon needs to plan a surgery by understanding the dimensions and profile of organ, 3D printing works well. Engineers can extract profile of the jaw from CT scan image and provide lifescale model of the jaw, as shown in Fig. 6.1. In a study, it was found that the surgeons modified surgery plan based on 3D printed models in a significant percentage of surgeries.

Also, these 3D models can be shown to the patient and the bystanders to get a better informed consent.

These models can further be used during training sessions.

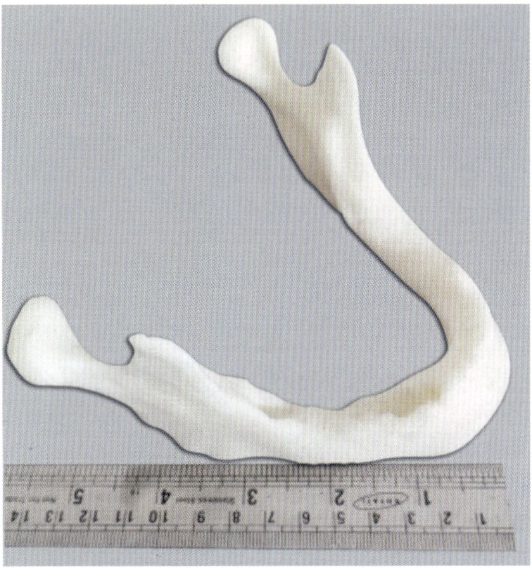

Fig. 6.1: A 3D model of jaw for orthognathic surgery

Patient-specific Implants

Metallic implants, mainly used in orthopaedic surgeries, come in standard sizes. Some patients may need implants in specific size and shape. For such a patient, an engineer can design the custom implant and get it 3D printed. Traditional manufacturing methods will cost hundreds time more for it.